Vegan Beauty Makeover

Reut Barak

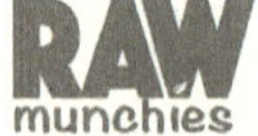

ISBN 9781793435705

TABLE OF CONTENTS

PREFACE

Hello, beautiful!
Welcome to your 30-day vegan beauty makeover.

In the following month, you are going to learn about yourself and your body.

- On day 1: You will get started by preparing the plan to have everything ready when you need it.
- On day 2: You will learn the technique of designing your own eyebrows in a way that fits your facial features, while looking healthy. You'll also make a smoothie recipe.

- On day 3: You will practice a relaxation exercise and get connected to your body, leaving you calm, optimistic, and confident. You will also make a healthy spiralized noodles recipe.
- On day 4: You will learn how to do skin brushing to increase your circulation and get naturally glowing skin.
- On day 5: You will learn how to improve your sleep and enjoy the advantages of this rest. You'll also get your first salad recipe.
- On day 6: You will learn how to take good care of your hair and get it to glow naturally.
- On day 7: You will do a special self-esteem building exercise to connect to the things you love about yourself, feel confident, learn how to be attractive and how to accept yourself the way you are. You'll also make a delicious smoothie.
- On day 8: You will learn how to identify toxins in cosmetics, and you will do a toxic-free makeover to your five makeup essentials.

- On day 9: You will learn about the benefits of fruit, enjoy a restful day, and make a loving fruit salad.
- On day 10: You will learn how to properly clean and file your nails.
- On day 11: You will learn a technique of stress release and get some of the things that trouble you out of the way. You will also make another wonderful smoothie.
- On day 12: You will learn the method of oil pulling to get clean and healthy teeth.
- On day 13: You will learn about the Chinese approach to wrinkles and how the lines reflect the inside of your body. You will also make amazing lettuce wraps.
- On day 14: You will enjoy a beautiful walk in nature and get exposed to fresh air and antioxidants to replenish your vitality.
- On day 15: You will do an exercise of rest and rejuvenation to gain focus in your thoughts and clear clutter from your mind.

- On day 16: You will learn about healthy food combinations, the best ways to time the different sugars, and get tips about juicing versus eating fruit whole.
- On day 17: You will do a dancing exercise that will release your inner spirit, and move all your muscles. You will also make another recipe of spiralized noodles.
- On day 18: You will learn how to declutter your wardrobe and keep the right clothes, so that when you open the closet door, you will be confident that you will always look your best.
- On day 19: You will learn how to choose new clothing items, that are a fit with the way you see yourself and the way you want to present yourself to the world. You will also get tips on how to accentuate your body and the accessories you wear.
- On day 20: You will learn about the four ways the body cleanses itself, and get introduced to the lymphatic system. You will also make another delicious salad.

- On day 21: You will learn about the effects of detox, what to expect when your body goes through a cleanse, and how to control detox using the pyramid of foods.

- On day 22: You will learn how to make your own essential oil blend, how to calculate oil dilution, and you will create your own scent stamp to use as both oil and fragrance. You will also make one last delicious salad.

- On day 23: You will have a makeup tutorial, where you'll learn how to accentuate your facial features and look your best, while maintaining a natural look.

- On day 24: You will learn the benefits of the different herbs that you can use on a daily basis, in your own kitchen, to strengthen the different systems of your body.

- On day 25: You will learn the special Magic Wand exercise which connects you to your inner desires and dreams, and reveals your true self, underneath the pressures of daily stress and routine.

You will also make a delicious raw
vegan soup.
- On day 26: You will learn about the
benefits and the rules of fasting and
complete the first of two days of a grape
fast.
- On day 27: You will learn more about
fasting, complete the grape fast, and do
a special writing exercise to connect to
your inner self.
- On day 28: You will increase your
kidney filtration and clean your body of
toxins by timing your foods.
- On day 29: You will have a delicious
smoothie, and a night out with friends
to flaunt your beautiful self and share
all that you've learned.
- On day 30: You will review all you've
achieved, make a great rewarding sushi
recipe, and celebrate your amazing
transformation.

Throughout the series, you will also be
introduced to expert resources you can use if you
want to know more about a certain subject, and
tips for further learning.

Are you ready?
Get set.
Go!

SHOPPING LISTS

ITEMS SHOPPING LISTS

- Day 1: Toxic-free soap and shampoo
- Day 2: A pair of tweezers
- Day 2: A hair comb with thin teeth
- Day 2: A blender or food processor to make smoothies
- Day 3: A spiralizer
- Day 4: A natural bristle skin brush
- Day 5: A bottle of 100% pure lavender oil
- Day 6: A detangle (wide-tooth) comb
- Day 6: Grapeseed carrier oil
- Day 8: Toxic-free cosmetics (cream, eyeliner, mascara, foundation and concealer, lipstick)
- Day 10: A nail file with a triangular tip or a cuticle pusher
- Day 12: Coconut oil
- Day 12: Baking soda (sodium bicarbonate)
- Day 19: A new item of clothing - more information on the day
- Day 22: Essential oils - more information on the day
- Day 30: Rolling mat for sushi

FOOD SHOPPING LISTS

Spices and for all recipes:

- rosemary
- tarragon
- oregano
- nutmeg powder
- paprika
- garlic powder
- ginger powder
- 5 spice
- chili flakes

Other ingredients for all recipes:

- cold-pressed olive oil
- coconut aminos
- Himalayan salt or sea salt
- alcohol-free vanilla extract
- cold-pressed sesame oil
- maple syrup
- apple cider vinegar
- almond extract
- coconut flakes

Fruit and vegetables for individual recipes with quantities:

Day 2: Daring Dill Smoothie:
- 1 cup dill
- 2 cucumbers
- 3 lemons
- ¼ cup mint

Day 3: Traditional Pesto Noodles:
- 6 zucchini
- 6 cups fresh basil leaves
- 1 ½ cups pine nuts
- ¾ cup walnuts

Day 5: Creative Colors of the Rainbow Salad:
- 1 avocado
- 1 tomato
- ½ yellow bell pepper
- ½ cauliflower
- ½ red cabbage
- 2 lemons
- 1 handful sunflower seeds

Day 7: Mega Morning Glory Smoothie:
- 3 cups strawberries

- 3 cups grapes
- 1 mango
- 1 apple
- 1 banana

Day 9: Magical Mango Berry Salad:

- 1 mango
- 1 cup blueberries
- 2 cups strawberries
- 6 bananas

Day 11: Dark Dream Smoothie:

- 1 cup blackberries
- 2 cups strawberries
- 6 bananas

Day 13: Lettuce Wraps:

- 10-12 large lettuce leaves
- ½ red pepper
- ½ cup chives
- 2 cups bean sprouts

Day 17: Fresh Style Pad Thai Noodles:

- 2 zucchini
- ½ cup chives
- ½ red bell pepper

- 1 lemon
- ½ tablespoon freshly grated ginger root
- 1 carrot
- 4 radishes
- 1 cup bean sprouts
- handful fresh coriander

Day 20: Amazing Asian Radish Salad:

- 2 cups radish
- 1 cucumber
- 1 avocado
- ¼ cup scallions
- 2 lemons
- ½ teaspoon freshly grated ginger root

Day 22: Magic Mediterranean Salad:

- 2 bell peppers in different colors
- 2 small cucumbers
- 2 tomatoes
- ½ onion
- 1 lemon

Day 25: Cream of Celery Soup:

- 6 long celery ribs
- ½ cup chopped dill
- 1 lemon

- chopped chives

Day 29: Precious Peach Smoothie:
- 5–6 peaches
- 1–2 cups strawberries
- the juice of 7 oranges

Day 30: Mega Sushi:
- 1 parsnip
- ½ lemon
- 1 teaspoon freshly grated ginger root
- 2 avocados
- ½ bell pepper
- ½ small cucumber
- 2–3 radishes
- 3–4 untoasted nori sheets
- sprinkle sesame seeds

DAY 1: GETTING STARTED

Hello, beautiful!

First, let me congratulate you on investing in yourself and in doing this amazing 30-day vegan beauty makeover transformation, to be the best you that you can be, beautiful from the inside out and shining because you are healthy and radiant.

This is the first day of the program and today you are going to get started by preparing for all the great days to come. When you come back home, you will treat yourself to a beautiful nourishing shower with your new toxic-free soap and shampoo from the list.

Are you ready?

Planning and getting started are the most important parts of any task, especially your own transformation. Everything else will depend on it.

You have some very important work today, to get all the things that you will need - both from the Items Shopping List and from the Food Shopping Lists - for the next few days. There are thirteen recipes in the book, and the list is sorted, with quantities, according to the days in which you will need the ingredients.

After you are done, you will get to come home and connect to your body and your beauty with a pampering, nourishing, natural-ingredients shower.

Showering with safe products:
Using toxic-free products is so important.
Our skin absorbs the chemicals we put on it and they go into the bloodstream. You will learn more about this on Day 8 (Safe Cosmetics) and Day 20 (Cleaning the Body). For now, let's focus on buying a good soap and a good shampoo.

As part of your shopping today, take a trip to the

local health shop, and ask them to let you look at toxic-free products for soap and shampoo. Ask them to give you products that don't have synthetic colors, fragrances, and preservatives, and make sure that the ingredients lists are mainly made of words you know, like "olive oil" or "citrus."

In the appendix section of this book, there is an alphabetical list of toxins found in cosmetics and hygiene products. Use it as a reference when you make your choice between the different options.

Time to go shopping! Go to page 15, where you will find the shopping lists. Allow yourself enough time to get all the items that you will need for the next few days. Don't forget the toxic-free soap and shampoo for today.

Done shopping?
Now comes the fun part.
Go back home and give yourself a nice warm shower, that leaves you feeling fresh and connected to your natural beauty. Massage yourself when you put the soap on. You've done an important task today and you deserve a treat!

I hope you've had a great day, getting started and also making the first step in reconnecting to your natural, gorgeous self. There's a lot of amazing things you are about to do in the month that follows.

Are you ready?

Tomorrow, you are going to make a deeper connection with your beauty, by designing your eyebrows in a way that makes your face look both natural and glamorous.

DAY 2: BEAUTIFUL EYEBROWS

Hello, beautiful!

First, let me congratulate you on completing the first day of the 30-day vegan beauty makeover and getting the things you need to get started.

This is the second day of the program and today, you are going to work on the first noticeable part of your face: the eyebrows. You also have your first new recipe, the Daring Dill Smoothie, which you will find at the end of the book, in the recipe section.

This eyebrow tutorial is going to be a very quick and easy one. It's actually a lot simpler than you think, and you can do it yourself. All you will need is:

- a mirror
- the thin side of a hair comb (or an eyebrow comb, if you have one)
- a good pair of tweezers

You're going to start by cleaning the eyebrows up a bit. First, you'll clean the middle part, at the top of the nose, between the eyebrows. This does not require a lot of delicacy and many women even do it with wax. Make sure you use good tweezers, and pull in the direction of the growth, getting each hair completely out.

Cleaning the area around the eyebrow:
First, you are going to clean the area above the eyebrow. Start by combing the eyebrows using the thin end of a hair comb, or an eyebrow comb. Then, remove any strays that don't go with a natural direction of the eyebrow.

Now, move to the sides of the eyebrows. Remove any stray hairs that grow below the eyebrows, on the sides of your eyes, and above the eyebrows. Also, remove hairs in the edges that make the eyebrow seem like it's closed inward and wraps around the eye.

So far, all you've done is intensify the eyebrows, by creating a very clear definition around them.

You might find that for you, this has been enough and just by having cleared the eyebrows, you now have the look that you desired.

When it comes to natural beauty, there's no need to do much.

Actresses like Keira Knightley, Denise Richards, and Emma Watson have been famous for their natural-looking, large eyebrows, and this type of beauty just might be exactly what you're looking for.

Shaping the eyebrows:
If you want to shape your eyebrows, first you must decide on the shape you are aiming for. The best tweezing creates a balanced appearance. There are three rules of thumb to remember:

- Avoid over-tweezing. Natural eyebrows have a certain thickness that gives the face an element of youthfulness. Over-tweezing might create an older, rigid appearance.
- The longer the face, the longer the

eyebrows should be.

- The rounder the face, the more angular the eyebrows should be.

There are many methods within these rules and the best tip is to think of the end result: would you like a soft appearance, or a more accentuated expression? Is there a celebrity whose face and skin tone are similar to yours and you like their eyebrow style? Did you get some good advice from an eyebrow expert which you would like to apply today?

Once you've decided on your desired change, proceed carefully. Every time you remove a hair or two, go back and look at the whole face, to make sure you're headed in the right direction.

Once you're done, give yourself a nice, warm face wash and dry with a soft towel.

If you liked today's exercise and want to know more about how to get great eyebrows, I highly recommend the Kindle e-book, *Naked Beauty*, by raw vegan beautician, Shakaya Leone. She used to work with celebrities, and she lists instructions and examples there.

I hope you had a great time today, and you feel

more connected to yourself and your beauty, with beautiful eyebrows to brighten up your look!

Okay, time for a treat! Head over to the recipe section and have a wonderful smoothie.

Tomorrow, you are going to make a deeper connection with your body by doing a relaxation exercise.

DAY 3: RELAXATION EXERCISE

Hello, beautiful!

First, let me congratulate you on completing the second day of the 30-day vegan beauty makeover and getting a beautiful look with freshly tweezed eyebrows.

This is the third day of the program and today you are going to connect to your inner beauty through a relaxation exercise. You also have a new recipe, the Traditional Pesto Noodles, which you will find at the end of the book, in the recipe section.

As we all know, stress takes a toll on the body, on how you look, sleep, digest your foods, absorb nutrients, and feel about yourself. This relaxation exercise is designed to release this tension and help you reconnect to a slower and more aware sensation.

It's best if you could take a couple of minutes and either sit on a comfortable chair, or lay down on a mattress, or a towel. You'll find that after a couple of times of doing this exercise, you'll be able to perform it on a busy bus, on the train, on the plane, in the middle of the day, and even standing in line to get your morning cup of tea.

Are you ready?

Once you've gotten comfortable, start by taking a deep breath.

Let the air in; give it a moment to settle. And now, let it go.

Let's do this again: let the air in, give it a moment to settle. And let it go.

One last time: let the air in, let it settle, and let it go.

Now, you're going to start by relaxing your toes. Your toes and your feet are the bottom part of your posture and carry your weight throughout the day.

So let's start by relaxing them. Just allow them to be as they want to be. In your mind, say to them, "Relax." You've probably immediately felt a release of your back and your neck.

Once you've felt the relaxation, you're going to move on.

Now, you'll relax the rest of the foot. Take your time. Make sure you've felt that release, that "ahh" moment of relaxation.

Once you've relaxed your feet, slowly move to your ankles. Take your time, very slowly.

When you're ready, gently move to your legs and relax them. You're probably feeling many other places are relaxing as you are doing this exercise, sometimes even internal organs - you might feel a nice feeling in your tummy, or your chest.

Now, slowly move up and start relaxing your knees, and then, the top part of your legs.

The next thing you're going to relax is your hands, your fingers. Those same fingers that allow you to do things are now going to a more passive mode.

When your fingers feel released, slowly move up your arms and relax them and then the elbows. Then, go all the way up to the shoulders and relax them too.

Release any stress in your neck. You can let your head fall forward a bit.

Once you've done your legs, arms, and neck, it's time to do the main part of your body.

You'll start with the tummy. Feel warmth and relaxation in the tummy. Everything is just flowing slowly. Take another deep breath and let it go. And one more breath. Let it go.

You will notice that this also relaxes your chest. Now, you'll move to the chest, and slowly relax any remaining tension there.

Now, you're just going to move on to your head. Softly relax all your facial muscles. Relax the area behind your ears. Release your jaw. Take a breath through your nose. You have all the time in the world. Close your eyes for a few seconds, and see if there is any tension in the body that you still want to release, and just let it go.

Now, observe your thoughts. Realize that all thoughts are optional. You can have any thoughts that you like. If there are any thoughts you don't like, you can easily watch them evaporate and release. Watch them move away from you until they are too far to see.

Close your eyes again for a few minutes. Be in this state of relaxation. Then, when you're ready, take one last deep breath, and go back to your day with bliss and optimism, flowing with relaxation, and feeling the beauty and grace of your body in every step and action you take.

Today's exercise was inspired by Osho's book, *Body Mind Balancing*. If you're interested in finding out more about relaxation exercises, and a different perspective of the body, this book is highly recommended.

I hope you had a great time today, and you feel more relaxed, flowing, and happy.

Okay, time for a treat! Head over to the recipe section and have a wonderful noodles recipe.

Tomorrow, you are going to make a deeper connection with your body with skin brushing for great circulation and beautiful glow.

DAY 4: BEAUTIFUL SKIN

Hello, beautiful!

First, let me congratulate you on completing the third day of the 30-day vegan beauty makeover and getting connected to your body through a deep relaxation exercise.

This is the forth day of the program and today, you are going to do dry skin brushing.

Your skin is your largest elimination organ, and skin care is one of the top priorities. Skin brushing is a great way to clear out old cells, increase circulation, and get beautiful, glowing skin. This is also beneficial for detox, as you'll discover on Day 20, when you learn about the four ways in and out of the body.

Skin brushing is a lot of fun.

It doesn't take long and leaves you feeling like you've just had a nice massage. All you will need is a natural bristle skin brush, a brush that is soft and kind to the skin, which is on the shopping list for today.

Okay, let's get started.

Start by brushing your feet. Use the brush gently, in a small circular motion. Continue, going upward, toward the knee of each leg, and then all the way up to the top of the leg until you've reached the thigh.

When you are done with the legs, it's time to move upward, to the arms. Start with the hands and slowly move, brushing the arms, toward the shoulders.

Once you're done with your legs and arms, it's time to move to the center of the body.

Start with your tummy. This time, go around the navel, in a clockwise direction, which is the direction in which our digestion works.

Move on to the chest and the rest of your front, and continue in small, circular motions. Then do the back.

Finally, do your shoulders and your neck. You

can do your face, but I would personally caution you, as this may be too harsh for the facial skin.

How did it feel?

You must now be feeling a bit warmer, and sensing a soft flow throughout the body.

If you want a bonus skin treatment, you can have a hot-and-cold shower following the skin brushing. This is a great way to increase the flow inside your body. The idea is to have a regular shower; then, at the end, turn the temperature down for a few seconds, then up again and repeat a few times. You don't have to do anything hard. Hot and cold doesn't mean freezing and boiling, of course. Just go for a little hotter and then a little colder, and repeat a few times.

I hope you had a great time today, getting beautiful fresh skin, and a feeling of flow through your body.

Tomorrow, you are going to make a deeper connection with your body by creating the space for a nourishing beauty sleep.

DAY 5: BEAUTY SLEEP

Hello, beautiful!

First, let me congratulate you on completing the fourth day of the 30-day vegan beauty makeover and rejuvenating your skin.

This is the fifth day of the program and today you are going to enhance your natural loveliness through beauty sleep. You also have a new recipe, the Creative Colors of the Rainbow Salad, which you will find at the end of the book, in the recipe section.

Sleep is so important. It is the part of the day in which the body has time to rebuild itself, to heal, and rejuvenate. Today, you are going to give yourself a special gift. In order to get that amazing beauty sleep, there are five things you are going to do.

1) Have fresh bedsheets:
It's always nice when the sheets are clean and tidy, smelling of a fresh wash, and the pillows are fluffed up, so start with making the bed.

2) Eat early:
Digestion is a vital part of health, and requires a lot of energy. You want to make sure that your body has completed this process and that during the night, it is no longer doing anything except for the processes that it must do during sleep. So today, make sure to finish your last meal very, very early. As early as five to six hours before you must go to bed, if you can. It's also best if you don't drink anything afterward, so that the whole system really gets a thorough rest.

3) Spread lavender oil on your pillow:
Lavender oil is a soothing essential oil, which will help you sleep strongly and it will take you less time to fall asleep.

You are going to sprinkle a little bit of lavender oil on your pillow, and then allow a few minutes for it to evaporate, and the scent to spread.

As we are using a pure, unblended oil, it will be very strong, so be careful to only use a few drops and do not put it directly on your skin.

4) Prepare so that you go to sleep early:
This is perhaps the most important part. Make sure you are going to sleep as early as you can. Our hormones are timed according to the sun, so going to sleep early will ensure you gain enough hours of deep sleep. Aim for around ten o'clock. This will make it easier for you to fall asleep naturally, and you won't risk getting over-exhausted. During the hour before you go to sleep, minimize your exposure to bright light and screens.

5) Use your wishes to feed your dreams:
Right before going to sleep tonight, close your eyes and think of three things that you want in your life. After that, breathe softly through your nose and believe in these things. See them happen.

I hope you have a great time today, preparing for your beauty sleep, and you feel freshness and inner strength tomorrow morning when you wake up. I wish you a wonderful night filled with beautiful dreams.

Okay, time for a treat! Head over to the recipe section and have a wonderful salad.

Tomorrow, you are going to take the beauty makeover one step further and do a lovely hair routine.

DAY 6: BEAUTIFUL HAIR

Hello, beautiful!

First, let me congratulate you on completing the fifth day of the 30-day vegan beauty makeover and getting nourishing, rejuvenating sleep. How did you feel this morning?

This is the sixth day of the program and today, it's all going to be about your hair. Your beautiful hair is one of the first things people notice about you when you walk down the street, glowing.

For today's hair routine, you will need a detangle comb. You're going to start by letting your hair loose, and slowly detangling it from the bottom up, using a detangle comb. A detangle comb is designed to have large gaps between the teeth so as to not break your hair. Work gently, especially if your hair is long, and go at a slow speed. Your hair is a macromolecule and will naturally detangle better when brushed slowly.

When you're done loosening any knots, you can use a regular comb, or even a thin comb to clean any dust or debris out of the hair.

Next, you are going to wash your hair. Make sure to use the toxic-free shampoo you bought to ensure no toxic chemicals get absorbed through the scalp. When you do this, give your scalp a loving massage. This will increase circulation and also clean your hair better. If you have to leave the house, make sure to give yourself enough time before you must go so that you can let your hair dry naturally, without using artificial heat, which can damage the hair.

Tonight, before you go to sleep, take half a tablespoon of grapeseed carrier oil and mix it with one drop of your lavender pure essential oil. Spread on the tips of your hair, and a bit on the lengths (but not on the scalp).

Allow your hair to absorb the oil. You will see the great results of moisture and shine when you wake up in the morning!

I hope you had a great time connecting to your beautiful, glowing hair.

Tomorrow, you are going to make a deeper connection with yourself, through a self-love and self-esteem building exercise.

DAY 7: SELF-LOVE

Hello, beautiful!

First, let me congratulate you on completing the sixth day of the 30-day vegan beauty makeover and walking around with glowing hair.

This is the seventh day of the program and today, you are going to find more self-love and self-esteem. You also have a new recipe, the Mega Morning Glory Smoothie, which you will find at the end of the book, in the recipe section.

Doing a self-esteem building exercise is a great way to reconnect to your inner desires, radiate confidence, and be naturally attractive.

Self-esteem and self-love are crucially important, no matter what you do. A woman who loves herself and takes good care of herself is always beautiful.

The biggest secret to self-esteem is that it is something we are born with. It's natural, but we forget this. We start talking to ourselves in limiting ways, and compare ourselves to external ideals. No animal in nature does this. When we were toddlers, we were proud of every step that we took on our own and of every little thing we made with our bare hands.

Today, you are going to remember this secret. Starting now. In the next exercise, you will write down the thoughts that come to mind, when you connect to the things you love and treasure about yourself.

Let's start.

Take a moment. Think of one thing that you are happy that you have. It could be your beautiful skin, or the depth of your eyes, or the style of your hair. One simple thing:

____

Now think of another thing, this time something from your personality. Perhaps you are clever, or make friends easily, are a great listener, or a good talker. Maybe you are very persuasive. Write it down.

____

Now, think of four skills that you are proud of. Are you good at teaching others, good at organizing; maybe you're a great cook, or a wonderful tennis player? Write these down.

____

____

____

Now, think of something that you love about your body. Perhaps you are very curvy, or tall, or have pretty hands, or maybe you have a beautiful voice. Write it down.

____

Now, think of something that you've done that makes you proud. Maybe it's a course you've done, a project you completed that was hard, a long distance walk, something you've made, an instrument you play or even a beautiful poem you wrote. Write it down.

Now, think of something that you have, that you really love and you are thankful for. Maybe it's a soft cushion to lay your head on at night, or a nice kitchen appliance that you like to use, your favorite dress, or the color of your wall. Something that is nice and relatable. Write it down.

Pause. Look at the things you've written. Realize that you are special. Nobody else gets to BE you. Everyone else only gets near. You are that person who is blessed with so many great things. Such potential! Only you have lived your life. Only you saw it from your eyes. There are things that only you know. This is what shaped your perspective. No one gets to live life the way you do.

Now, think of ten things that you are thankful for. This could be anything. This time, let your thoughts pour freely. Write them down.

____

____

____

____

____

____

____

____

Tonight, right before you go to sleep, think of these things. Take each one of them separately, and say, "I am grateful for..." and say it as you've listed it just now.

Now, think of three things that you love to do. Write them down.

____

____

____

These things you've just thought of are your talents. That's why you love doing them. Treasure them. They are what make you special.

Be confident in what you do. See how radiant you become, once you say, "I know what I'm doing." See how people are drawn to you.

The secret of self-love is acceptance; it's seeing your own light, without comparison. Decide, that from now on, you will be the point of reference. The rest of the world will just do their own thing, in their own way. You will keep doing the things that you love, without needing to explain anything, or ask any questions.

And since the secret to self-love is acceptance, now think of one thing you didn't always love about yourself. Something you wanted to change.

———————————————

Focus on that thing, and instead of wanting to change it, love yourself with it. Think of yourself with it. Think of how this actually makes you complete. There's nothing to fix here. You are perfect just the way you are.

Today, after you've taken a shower, look in the mirror, and say to yourself:

"Beauty is in the eye of the beholder. My opinion counts more than everyone else's. I now decide that I am the ideal. This is the definition of beauty. There are many types of perfect and this one is mine."

I wish you a wonderful day, filled with radiant self-love and confidence. Let's end with a great quote from the famous Casanova, one of the most attractive men of his time: "Be the flame, not the moth."

Okay, time for a treat! Head over to the recipe section and have a wonderful smoothie.

Tomorrow, you are going to learn about using safe cosmetics.

DAY 8: SAFE COSMETICS

Hello, beautiful!

First, let me congratulate you on completing the seventh day of the 30-day vegan beauty makeover and boosting your radiant self.

This is the eighth day of the program and today, you are going to do a toxic-free makeover for your cosmetics bag.

This is extremely important. The skin absorbs the chemicals we put on it, and they go into the bloodstream (just like the nicotine patch or the birth control patch). The skin also clears toxins out of the body, through sweating, so keeping it healthy and clear is important to overall wellness.

Because of this, when you put something on your skin, you want it to be as clean as the food you eat (if you can't eat it - don't put it on your skin).

So now, let's go on to detoxing your cosmetics. You're going to do this in two steps:

Step 1) Changing the Essentials.

The basic makeup ingredients are:
1. cream
2. eyeliner
3. mascara
4. foundation
5. concealer
6. a lip product (like a lipstick, which can also be used as blush)

The first step is to get these six products from absolute natural sources. This will ensure that your daily routine is a safe one. Eventually, you would want to go all the way and switch the rest of your makeup as well.

Today, you are going to go shopping for safe

makeup. What is safe makeup? Safe makeup products don't cause toxic chemicals to accumulate in your body. The best places to get them are either in health food shops, or online.

Here are the things you want to look out for:
- Words you cannot pronounce: you want most of the ingredients in the product to be things you already know, like "olive oil", "citrus," "cocoa powder," "aloe vera," or "aqua" (which means water). Words with ten letters or more, and a number, are usually manufactured chemicals.
- Synthetic colors and fragrances (often called "Parfum").
- Preservatives.

In the appendix section of the book, you'll find an alphabetical list of toxins found in makeup, compiled from different resources that specialize in tracking chemicals in cosmetics. It's always best to keep looking up toxins online on a regular basis, because new chemicals are introduced every day.

"Natural" and "Pure":
Did you know that the words "natural" and "pure" have no legal definition? This means that a

company can write these words on any product, even if it contains heavy toxins.

"Vegan" only means there are no animal-based ingredients, but there could still be heavily manufactured lab chemicals in the product.

The word "organic," on the other hand, is legally binding and means the ingredient was inspected to test it is organic.

Step 2) Changing the Rest of Your Makeup.

Decide that, from now on, every time that something runs out, you will buy the replacement from a natural source. Keep switching your makeup kit until it has a complete beauty makeover.

I hope you have a great time today, shopping for new cosmetics and also feel you've learned how to take great care of your beautiful skin and your body.

Tomorrow, you will have a true taste of detoxing, cleansing foods. Literally.

DAY 9: A LOVING DETOX SALAD

Hello, beautiful!

First, let me congratulate you on completing the eighth day of the 30-day vegan beauty makeover and giving your makeup a makeover.

This is the ninth day of the program and today, you have a treat: the wonderful Magical Mango Berry Fruit Salad, which you will find in the recipe section at the end of the book. It's got bananas, mango, strawberries, and blueberries... Yum!

You deserve this treat. You have been working so hard for the past eight days, and you must already see and feel the results. So now, it's time to take a rest and connect to the essence of fruit.

The Importance of Fruit:
Fruit are your best friends, and by fruit, we also mean the non-sweet ones like tomatoes, cucumbers, lemons, and peppers. They grow on plants, bear seeds, and have a high water content. This is what your body loves the most. Fruit are the most nutrient-dense foods, and the easiest to digest.

As humans, we are a frugivore species, like apes, (that eat bananas). Of course, if you take an ape away from its natural habitat, it would eat anything, but fruit is its favorite.

The Importance of Vegetables:
In today's world, where many of us live in colder countries, we eat food from the supermarket which has gone through refrigeration and other processes that deplete the nutrients. For this reason, adding vegetables is important, but the basis is still fruit.

You'll notice that in today's salad, there are only sweet ingredients. This is because we are separating the different types of sugars, and we're also eating the fruit whole. On Day 16, you'll learn about good food combinations.

Okay. Now, it's time to make this great treat, and have a beautiful, tasty fruit salad for a happy tummy!

Okay, time for a treat! Head over to the recipe section and have a salad.

I hope you have a great time making it, and you feel energetic and vibrant after it's complete.

Tomorrow, you are going to do some work on beautifying your nails.

DAY 10: BEAUTIFUL NAILS

Hello, beautiful!

First, let me congratulate you on completing the ninth day of the 30-day vegan beauty makeover and celebrating your achievement with an amazing treat of a fruit salad.

This is the tenth day of the program and today, you are going to take great care of your nails with easy nail shaping.

As you eat more healthy foods and cultivate healthy habits, you'll notice many changes in your body. One of them would be stronger, naturally shiny nails.

The secret to naturally healthy, strong nails is knowing that our nails are made of many layers. This means that the filing needs to be gentle.

1) Cleaning Your Nails:
Start by removing any chemicals that are coating the nail and then give your hands a good wash. Dry your hands and make sure your nails are dry, before you go to the next step.

2) Nail Shaping – Filing the Sides:
Carefully, start filing a nail from one side, working toward the middle. File only in one direction, as going back and forth would damage the delicate layers and can cause them to break. When doing the side, position the file parallel to the nail. If you are looking to create an oval shape, file at an angle.

Now file the same nail, from the other side, going inward again.

3) Nail Shaping – Filing the Middle:
Choose a direction in which to file the middle of the nail, and continue, only in that direction.

4) Cleanup:

When you are done shaping the nail, carefully insert the tip of the file, or a cuticle pusher, under the nail and moving slowly across the edge, expose any leftover nail layers. File these too. Lastly, position the file right at the edge of the nail, and file this edge downward lightly.

5) A nice massage:

When you are done repeating this process with all your nails, give your hands a nice refreshing massage using olive oil and mashed avocado. Then wash with natural soap.

How was it? Are you loving the new look and fresh, moist skin? I hope you had fun and that this quick tutorial has left you with shining, beautiful nails shaped as you like.

Tomorrow, you are going to take one step further on your internal path and release some stress.

DAY 11: STRESS

Hello, beautiful!

First, let me congratulate you on completing the tenth day of the 30-day vegan beauty makeover and getting beautiful, shining nails.

This is the eleventh day of the program and we are going to release some stress. You also have a new recipe, the Dark Dream Smoothie, which you will find at the end of the book, in the recipe section.

Stress is one of the worst environmental impacts on your health, beauty, and your ability to deal with what's in front of you. If you add stress to any problem, it grows.

Most problems actually have a simple solution, or a form of inner acceptance, once the stress is removed. On day 3, you did a relaxation exercise; today you'll go one step further and eliminate the causes of tension, leaving you feeling more relaxed, flowing, loving, and focused. You're going to start by picking three things that stress you and writing them down:

1) Something big:

The first stress you will write down needs to be something that really bothers you, that makes you say to yourself, "If I could solve this one thing, I'd feel like I've gone on vacation." Think of something that really affects your life and write it down:

____

____

Doesn't it feel good to have put it down on paper?

Part of what makes something a lot more stressful than it can be is the fact that we look away from it. It is so daunting to us that we don't want to think about it.

Unfortunately, we can't look away for long, and this creates a lot of worry and even more stress. It makes the thing look a lot larger than it is. Say, for example, you must find a new home, or you are starting a new job. Doesn't it feel a lot easier once you've signed the lease, or had your first day? Even though you still don't know how things will really turn out in the end, just having some clarity helps.

2) Something annoying:

There are different types of stress. Sometimes something does not affect your life dramatically. Instead, it's there all the time and you keep having to deal with it. Think of something you'd really like to just eliminate and write it down:

____

____

3) Something frightening, but exciting:

For the third stress, pick something that you want to do, but that makes you feel fear; something that's important for you to do. This can be a new project you're starting, or something you always wanted to learn, or even a speech or a video you wanted to make and it gives you stage fright. Write it down:

____

____

This kind of stress is not like the other ones. This one is actually positive; it's more like too much excitement. This is why you're going to start with this one. List three reasons why you haven't done this yet, or why it causes you stress when you do it.

One of them needs to be completely silly (like a fear that something completely irrational would go wrong). Write them down:

____

____

____

Now, write down the worst-case scenario. What is the worst thing that could happen if you did complete this activity all the way? How bad could it possibly be? Write this down:

____

____

____

____

Seems unlikely, right? It's such a relief to see that most of the fear is just in the head. Now, imagine that you did do it all, just like you want to, and it went great. How would that feel? Write down 3 emotions:

____

____

____

Feels lighter, doesn't it? This one thing you really want now seems a lot more reachable, easier.

Okay, now you're going to go back to number 2, "Something annoying."

Here you're going to use your sense of humor.

Imagine a funny way, like divine intervention, or something ridiculous that happens and completely solves this one annoying stress. Write this down:

____

____

____

____

Great. Now, ask yourself, what exactly about this situation that you have to deal with is getting on your nerves? Avoid the common answers of "it just is," or "things like that are always annoying." You already know this; now you're trying to go beyond the obvious layer of the problem. So why is this bothering you? Write this down:

____

____

____

____

Now, you're going to go into the future. A year from now, in a realistic way, this stress got resolved. What happened? How did circumstances change to eliminate the problem? Write this down:

____

____

____

____

Now, let's be proactive. Write down one thing that you can do this week or next week that would make this situation better for you:

____

____

____

____

Now, after you've done stress-exciting and stress-annoying, you're going to do stress-anxiety, the big problem you wrote down in number 1.

Do you know someone who had a similar problem and solved it? Maybe you need to look online to find them. Who was that person?

Say you want to find love. Did you know that there is a TED Talk by a woman who reverse-engineered her search on an online dating site, and went from being the least noticeable girl to the most popular woman online, and found the one man she was waiting for? You can look her up. Her name is Amy Webb.

Say it's finances or education that stress you. Did you know that Liz Murray, who was homeless, made her way back to school, got a scholarship, and graduated from Harvard?

Janette Murray-Wakelin decided to treat her highly aggressive breast cancer, with six months left to live, through a fully raw lifestyle and natural treatments. Years later, she's completed 366 consecutive marathons around Australia.

Temple Grandin did not cure her autism...she did get a PhD, and is a world-known lecturer on both her subject and on autism.

Who solved your big problem? Write down their name:

____

Now it's your turn. Break your problem into three parts that make it difficult. For example, if you're looking for an apartment, your three components can be prices in the market, how close you want to be to your job or to schools, and availability of apartments right now.

Write down the three most important components of your problem.

____

____

____

____

And now for the action. This week, you are going to spend at least two hours educating yourself on this issue. It could be reading a book, or watching a lecture by someone who's solved it. It could be chatting to an expert who can guide you, or finding a mentor with experience who could lead you on how to better solve it.

Feeling better already?

I hope you had a great time today, dealing with the things that stress you from an empowered and confident perspective, and feeling more in tune with yourself and more relaxed.

Okay, time for a treat! Head over to the recipe

section and have a wonderful smoothie.

Tomorrow, you are going to make a deeper connection with your body by doing an oil pulling exercise, to get healthy, clean teeth.

DAY 12: BEAUTIFUL TEETH

Hello, beautiful!

First, let me congratulate you on completing the eleventh day of the 30-day vegan beauty makeover and empowering yourself to deal with stresses.

This is the twelfth day of the program and today, you're going to do some oil pulling. Oil pulling is a great, easy way to get your teeth clean. All you'll need is the coconut oil, which is on the shopping list for today, two teaspoons, and two bowls.

This will take about twenty minutes, so make sure you are alone in a room and won't be disturbed.

To begin, place some oil from the jar into one of the bowls using a teaspoon. Then, using another teaspoon, take some of that oil into your mouth and start swirling it. Swirl, swirl, swirl. When you feel too much moisture has accumulated, spit it into the second bowl and then take fresh oil to swirl. Continue for about twenty minutes, as doing this a long period of time helps alkalize the mouth.

Never swallow this oil, as it contains the toxins you've been cleansing. When you are done, dispose of it in a bag and brush your teeth with baking soda.

How did that feel?

You must have a sensation of freshness now, since you've just spent twenty minutes stimulating your gums and alkalizing your saliva.

You can do this with different natural oils, other than coconut oil, but fruit-based ones are best.

Want a bonus? You can also use a water flusher to remove any unwanted dirt that's been accumulated on your teeth over time.

If you liked this and you'd like to know more about today's oil pulling, you might be interested in looking up the case of Christie Aphrodite, who's cured cavities and gum problems using this method.

I hope you had a great time today, and you feel more confident with your clean and beautiful teeth.

Tomorrow, you are going to make a deeper connection with your body by understanding wrinkles, their causes and elimination.

DAY 13: SMOOTHING WRINKLES

Hello, beautiful!

First, let me congratulate you on completing the twelfth day of the 30-day vegan beauty makeover and getting bright and beautiful teeth.

This is the thirteenth day of the program and today, you're going to learn three valuable insights on wrinkles. Right after this chapter, there is an interview with Dr. Robert Morse about anti-aging. He's a nutritionist who has helped people in their eighties and nineties get wrinkle-free skin. You also have a new recipe, of Lettuce Wraps, which you will find at the end of the book, in the recipe section.

Ever wondered why every person has wrinkles in different places, and some don't have them at all? Here is a learning exercise. Go to Google and type in "Chinese face map." Look at the images. You will notice something surprising: the areas of our face are representative of our inner organs!

Isn't this a great revelation? This means that by curing and purifying both the inner part of ourselves and our skin, we can have a radiant, wrinkle-free, glowing face. It also means that through wrinkles, we can know what is going on inside the body real-time. The mirror is giving you a wonderful way of knowing what's going on!

I'll share a little secret with you: I get laugh lines the day after I eat nuts. This is because that area of the face corresponds with a part of my digestive system that is sensitive to nuts.

Today, you will learn to look at wrinkles from three perspectives: the skin itself, the different parts of the body that effect how your facial skin looks, and the body as a whole.

1) The skin itself:

This is probably the most intuitive. The skin itself needs to be in a healthy condition. At the end of this chapter, you will get a natural skin alkalization exercise.

2) The different parts of the body that effect how your facial skin looks:

Certain elements are consistent across the different Chinese face maps. For example, kidneys and adrenal glands are represented in the area under and around the eyes, the liver between the eyebrows, and the digestive system is around the mouth.

You can use this knowledge. Start by taking a good look in the mirror and note what you see.

Write down three areas you would like to work on the most. Which parts of your body need strengthening?

____

____

____

On Day 24, you will learn how to work with herbs to strengthen and rebuild tissue. Another good source of herbs are herbal formulas. I like to learn from the ingredients lists in the formulas by Dr. Morse, who has helped eighty-year-old patients to have vibrant, wrinkle-free skin. You can read a bonus interview with him, right after this chapter.

3) The body as a whole:

Good skin begins with overall good health and good circulation, alkalization, and hydration. Eating healthy, fresh, whole foods and making sure to get good quality air and regular movement are key to ensuring the body gets sufficient circulation, alkalization, and hydration (notice that we didn't list water here, as the amount of liquids you need to drink depends highly on the climate you live in and the type of activities you do).

Now, to the skin exercise for the day.

First of all, why not have another go at skin brushing (see Day 4)? This is a very beneficial activity for your entire body.

After you're done, give your face a nice cleansing rinse. Then, mash a little bit of banana (you can do this with a fork or with your fingers) and spread a thin layer of it over your face. Massage it so that it's absorbed well in the skin. Banana is like a natural soothing cream. It's dense in nutrients and alkalizing.

Leave the cream on for at least twenty minutes. This is easy to do, since the color is completely clear, making the cream invisible. When you are done, rinse well and take a good look in the mirror. You will be surprised at the change!

I hope you feel you've learned a natural, new and modern approach to skin care and understanding your body, and that you feel great and confident.

Okay, time for a treat! Head over to the recipe section and have wonderful lettuce wraps.

Tomorrow, you are going to make a deeper connection with your body by taking a walk in nature.

AN INTERVIEW WITH DR. ROBERT MORSE

Interview with Dr. Robert Morse, Doctor of Naturopathy and Biochemistry, herbalist and iridologist. This interview was edited from the original recording, with the approval of Dr. Robert Morse. The original recording can be found at: http://rawmunchies.org/dmi/

Hi and welcome to the Vegan Beauty Makeover. Today we have an amazing treat—a quick interview with Dr. Robert Morse, Doctor of Naturopathy and Biochemistry, herbalist and iridologist.

You have seen over 250,000 patients in hospitals and clinics, have saved people who had just a few weeks left to live, and restored them to full health, which is amazing!!! But what surprised me when I first read your book and got introduced to this lifestyle, is that it anti-ages. And you've seen cases of getting rid of wrinkles with people in their 80s and 90s, and had mid-aged patients get their natural hair color back.

Oh, yes. Absolutely.

So...what's your secret? What makes people anti-age, and more importantly, what makes us sick in the first place?

Okay, so think about this: there are only two sides of chemistry, right? And when you look at the world, it's dualistic. Creation is dualistic—there's only two sides to it. So when you look at chemistry, there's two sides to it: one is well known as the acid side, especially in the health field, and the other side is the base side, or we call it alkaline side.

When you take a look at what breaks things down, like tissues, and makes a hair gray and dehydrates and all that... that's always the acid side of chemistry.

The alkaline side of chemistry is your electrolytes—it hydrates you.

Both sides don't have the same effect—they have opposite effects.

In chemistry, the acid side of chemistry is dehydrating, and they call this side cationic, which means it's corrosive, but it's agglomerating, meaning things get hard, stiff and tight.

You can feel that in your body. When you work out, sometimes you get stiff and hard. That's from acidosis—that's from creating all this activity, and activity creates more metabolism. Metabolic waste in the human body is acidic.

Well...when you take a look at foods, foods fall in the same category. There's a bunch of foods that are acid forming and there are certain foods that are alkaline forming. Man just loves the acid-forming foods! When you look at it, man eats predominantly acid-forming foods: that's your proteins, your beans, your grains, your cooked dairy products, and cheeses. And then, on top of that, your body creates several pounds of acid waste from metabolism. So, when you combine the two, people are just living in the acidic world. Then, the air is getting acidic from all the by-products, and manufacturing, and cars... things are getting more and more acidic. Well, that's corrosive; that's inflammatory. Inflammation ranges in people all over the place, and then, of course, the kidneys shut down and tumors form and things like that.

That's what creates the wrinkles, because when you're acidic, that's corrosive and destroying to tissue, so then the body has to do something to fight that, and if it's not in the diet, then it has to take it out of the body.

The number one constituent that the body takes and uses is calcium. A lot of the great universities around the world have discovered the calcium buffering system, which means that the body steals calcium out of its connective tissue and skeletal tissue to fight all this acidosis.

When that happens, you get bruising easy, you get varicose and spider veins, your skin wrinkles, you get prolapses. With a lot of women, their uterus prolapses, bladders prolapse, bowels prolapse...your skin and your eyelids. Everything starts getting weak, because the body is borrowing that calcium. It's kind of like a mother who has a parathyroid weakness, doesn't utilize calcium in her own diet, doesn't even have it in her diet, and then she has a baby. That baby start stealing all her calcium. Then her teeth disintegrate, her bones disintegrate, because the baby needs the calcium. Of course, there's only one place to get it if it isn't in the diet.

So, when you take a look at that, fruits, berries, and melons, and salads are your alkaline-forming foods. Your beans, your grains, your pasteurized and processed foods are all acid-forming foods, and man lives predominantly on acid-forming foods. And so, he gets more and more acidic. You get pain, you get swelling, you get tumors, you get arthritis. All the diseases that medical doctors speak of are all in the world of acidosis.

So, how do you cure people? What do you do?

You walk on to the other side of chemistry. That's how simple it is.

You cannot get well by continuing down the acid side, because you'll see the same thing, but worse and worse and worse... When you go to the other side of chemistry, you're now on the electrolytes, on the hydrating side of chemistry, the anionic environment. Now your body starts hydrating and rebuilding itself.

I went, as you were talking, on raw foods. They're not processed. You've got fruits and berries and melons, which are more homosapien foods, and then you get some salads, but those are herbivore foods. The body starts hydrating and repairing itself.

You see that every time. I could take a case, let's say of Lou Gehrig's or MS, that's in a wheelchair, they have brain lesions, they can't talk anymore, they can't walk; of course, they start getting muddled. That is a high state of acidosis. You can get them on the other side, into a high level electrically of fruits and berries and melons, give them a few herbs to repair things, and pretty soon they're up walking, talking, and having a life again.

Amazing!

And we've done that years and years and years.

That's amazing. And I think what surprises us is that this knowledge is not more prevalent.

It should be, because it's very simple: there are only two sides of chemistry. Pick one. Each side has its own effect upon you. Just studying a little of that shows you which side you should be on.

Well, understanding a little bit about the food you eat helps a great deal to kind of close your case for you. Especially when you look at humans; they're frugivores. So, a human is not a paleo: he's not a protein eater; he doesn't have hair all over him for cold climate survival. He's an islander. And man originated as an islander—homosapiens originated as an islander species, a primate-ish species.

When you move your diet to the high (fruits, berries, and melons), the body starts cleaning and regenerating. The nervous system rebuilds. The liver rebuilds and cleans itself. All these things start rebuilding themselves.

When you see fatty livers, and all types of inflammatory problems, and lupus and Lymes, they can talk all day long about diseases, but in reality, it's all the state of acidosis in different locations and different degrees.

You can fix it all by walking on the other side of chemistry.

DAY 14: CONNECTING TO NATURE

Hello, beautiful!

First, let me congratulate you on completing the thirteenth day of the 30-day vegan beauty makeover and learning to get great-looking skin.

This is the fourteenth day of the program and today, you are going to do a little nature walk.

There are a lot of advantages to being out in the fresh air, with antioxidants and peace and quiet. And it's great to get out of the house and do something active. It's relaxing, and a wonderful way to move your body, exercise your limbs, and make sure you are moving toxins out of your system.

Today's walk will be a nice calming one. It doesn't even have to be long, just enough to get you to feel connected to nature.

Whether you're going to do this for 20 minutes or a full hour or even longer than that, the important part of the walk is to be very conscious of how you feel physically.

If you are too busy, don't worry. You don't have to do it all in one go. Maybe there's a small reserve next to you and you can walk there for five minutes at a time, a few times during the day.

Really relax and connect. Let the walk take you where it wants, without too much planning. If, on the way, you see a nice place, like a pretty bench to sit on, or a trail you'd like to follow, do so. Try the relaxation exercise from Day 3. See how different your walk feels after that.

Be sure to appreciate the beauty around you. This is immortal beauty. It was there long before us and will be there long after. That's why you feel beautiful when you are out in nature. You are always part of nature, and this is a good reminder of it. Like dolphins and penguins, you, too, are always beautiful.

Be aware of how walking feels, how your body moves and is charged from the inside. Walk at a comfortable pace and feel the ground under your feet. If it's warm and safe, try walking barefoot for a few minutes and feel the earth and rocks, or the sand under your feet.

Connect to the sounds, as well as to the silence. Listen to the singing of the birds, or the rustling of the trees. See if you can spot some animals that you don't normally see.

Try not to think. Especially not about things that worry you. If you are going with a friend, agree to walk in silence most of the time, and not get into too many conversations that might distract you from what you are experiencing and seeing.

Put the phone on silent.

I wish you have a great time during your walk today, and you end up feeling more connected to your body and your beauty, through fresh air and natural sensations.

Tomorrow, you are going to have a restful day to find peace and rejuvenation.

DAY 15: REST AND REJUVENATION

Hello, beautiful!

First, let me congratulate you on completing the fourteenth day of the 30-day vegan beauty makeover and getting your body nourished and vibrant through a beautiful walk in nature.

This is the fifteenth day of the program and today, you are going to rest.

That's right. It's exactly the middle of the program, and it's time to look proudly at everything you've done so far, and take a day of rest.

If you had a fairy godmother, who could magically make all your tasks and all your projects complete, what would you do? What is the thing that you have been waiting for? Is it a book you've been waiting to read, a friend you wanted to catch up with, a date night, a meditation exercise? What would you do once you've freed up your time?

Schedule one hour today in which you will not be disturbed. Then, find a comfortable chair or a mattress, and for twenty minutes, just do nothing. You can use the relaxation exercise you've learned or your own breathing or meditation exercise.

Do something that sets your mind free.

Another way to relax is simply to listen, to just hear the noises around like they are the music of the world. Take them in, like a symphony, without focusing on any particular sound.

Release your thoughts.

If a thought comes up, treat it like watching a bus. It came and now it goes away; there's no need to respond to it.

After you've relaxed, for the rest of the hour, do one or two things you've been waiting to do. If it's a catch up, call your friend; a date night, call and book a restaurant for later; a book you've been waiting to read, start reading it now. Treat yourself.

I hope you had a restful day today, and connected to some of the things you've been waiting to do.

Tomorrow is a very important day. You will learn about foods that go together and how to time your sugars and nutrients, so that your body is nourished and beautiful from the inside out.

DAY 16: FOODS THAT GO TOGETHER

Hello, beautiful!

First, let me congratulate you on completing the fifteenth day of the 30-day vegan beauty makeover. You've officially reached the middle of the program. Well done!

This is the sixteenth day of the program, and today you're going to learn about food combinations.

Good food combining is very important. It times the sugars right, and affects how much energy you have throughout the day. It's very easy to do, if you separate the foods into three groups:

1. Melons
2. Other sweet fruit
3. Everything else, separating proteins and starches

Group 1) Melons:

Melons (like melon, watermelon, cantaloupe, and papaya) are the fastest digesting of all foods.

Combining them with slower digesting foods would cause a delay in the process, and hold fruit sugars in the stomach while they ferment, causing alcohol levels in the blood to rise.

It's very important to wait half an hour after eating melons, to allow them time to digest.

Group 2) Other sweet fruit:

The next food group is the sweet fruit - for exactly the same reasons. Waiting at least half an hour after eating sweet fruit for these quick sugars to digest allows the stomach to finish the process and be ready for the next meal.

Within sweet fruit, some people also like to separate the more acidic fruit (like berries, citrus, sour fruits, and pineapple) from the more sweet ones (like bananas, dates, and raisins).

Group 3) Everything else, and separating proteins and starches:

After you've separated melons and sweet fruits, what remains is the slower digestive foods, like vegetables. These require at least one hour of waiting after eating them, and before eating the fast-digesting foods.

Within this group, it's important to separate proteins and starches. Of course, both should not be eaten with sweet fruit or melons.

Proteins, including nuts, need to be broken into amino acids. This requires hydrochloric acid to release pepsin. That produces an acidic-chemistry environment in the stomach.

Starches, like corn, quinoa, cereals, rice, and potatoes (if you're eating cooked foods) are the opposite. Their digestion requires alkaline digestive enzymes. That produces a base-chemistry environment in the stomach.

Okay, so you've just learned the easy separation into three food groups.

Another quick rule remains about sugars: Eat

your fruits and juice your vegetables.

Many people find the fiber in sweet fruit and melons important, because it helps with sugar metabolism. Juicing removes this fiber, so (unless you are on a juice fast) it is better to eat fruit whole.

With vegetables, on the other hand, juicing makes digestion easier, because of the high cellulose content in the vegetables.

Sugar worries? One last note:

Everything we eat has sugars. The important thing is to eat the simple ones (like the ones in fruit), combine and time them right, and avoid the more complex ones (like those in animal products and processed starches).

I hope you feel you've learned something today that makes you feel more in control of what you put into your body, and helps you eat in a way that makes your tummy happy.

Tomorrow, you are going to make a deeper connection with your body by doing a wild dance.

DAY 17: A LOVING DANCE

Hello, beautiful!

First, let me congratulate you on completing the sixteenth day of the 30-day vegan beauty makeover and getting valuable knowledge on sugars.

This is the seventeenth day of the program and today, you're going to do something fun: dance and feel happy with the body. You also have a new recipe, the Fresh Style Pad Thai Noodles, which you will find at the end of the book, in the recipe section.

Loving your body from the inside, and celebrating it, is so important. This is a great exercise and might feel a little bit adventurous to you, maybe even a bit naughty.

It only takes five minutes. Of course, you can always do it for more. So, let's get started:

Pick a song that makes you want to dance.

Then, find a room where nobody can see or hear you - it's probably best if you could do this using earphones.

And then...go wild! Play the music loudly. Really get into it. Do it ugly! Don't worry about how it looks. Shake your butt in all directions. Shake everything else. Throw your hands around. Kick your legs. Have you ever seen toddlers shake when they try to dance? That's what you're going for. Shake shake shake shake!

Dance for real, without any pretty movements, without being a dancer. You're not here to impress anyone! If you're alone, sing along loudly. Don't worry about the neighbors - it's just one song.

This is your own private party. Go mad. Dance like a wild caveman, with drums and fire. Imagine people are clapping for you, for being the craziest dancer gold medalist of the year.

Enjoy it.

You'll see how much energy is inside you, waiting to come out. Feel it bubbling through you, and move to the beat.

I hope you have a great time dancing to the rhythm of your own body, and you feel happy, energetic, and more connected to yourself and your beauty.

Okay, time for a treat! Head over to the recipe section and have a wonderful noodles recipe.

Tomorrow, you are going to do a closet makeover so you feel more confident when you present your beautiful self to the world.

DAY 18: LOVING YOUR CLOTHES

Hello, beautiful!

First, let me congratulate you on completing the seventeenth day of the 30-day vegan beauty makeover and connecting with your body and your inner soul through dance.

This is the eighteenth day of the program and today and tomorrow, you're going to do a wardrobe makeover.

Dressing is one of the most important things that you do every single day. It starts when you stand in front of your mirror and decide how you want to display yourself to the world. Dressing is about being seen, about creating an outfit that's beautiful and makes you feel empowered.

Today, you're going to do the first step of the wardrobe makeover. After this, you will have a closet that you love to open, and clothes that you can't wait to wear.

Are you ready?

There are many ways to reorganize the wardrobe. Some people say, "If you haven't worn something for a long period of time, throw it away." But sometimes, those clothes, that you haven't worn for a while, have sentimental value. Maybe it's that dress that you bought for an occasion, and seeing it reminds you of that night. Maybe it's the pants you bought for your previous job, that don't suit this one, but still look great. You keep these items because you love them. You might wear them again, and you might not, but that's not what's important.

What's important is to sort your clothes based on what makes you happy to have in your closet.

Let's get started.

Go to your closet and get all the clothes that you wear on a regular basis: the everyday shirts, trousers, jeans, skirts, socks, underwear, sweaters, coats, and dresses. All the clothes that you use to display yourself to the world on a regular basis, for work, for meeting friends, for fun, for sports.

Get all of them out of the closet and lay them on the bed or the couch in one pile. It's great to finally see what you have, right?

Now, pick each item. One at a time. Touch it and try to feel inside. When you hold it in your hands, does it make you really happy? Is there something about the fabric, something about the color, something about how it feels to have it, that really makes you delighted?

If it does, keep it.

If it doesn't, then it's had its time.

It's that easy. Sorting out and eliminating becomes easy once you realize that you don't have to do it based on how long you've owned something or how frequent you wear it, only by how much you love it.

There are many reasons why it's time to let an item go, and often it's difficult, even when it's the right thing to do.

Maybe you've just bought it. In the shop, it looked really nice under the fitting room spotlight, but now back at home it's not what you really want. That's okay. You've given it all the attention it wanted. Now it wants to go back to the shop and get refunded, so that it could find its rightful owner.

Just because you bought it doesn't mean you have to keep it.

You're not insulting the item.

If it was a present, don't worry. You are not insulting your friends either. No one would want you to keep something that doesn't make you really, really happy, right?

When you open your closet, you want to see only clothes that make you go, "Wow! I love wearing this! I love how this makes me feel." So don't feel bad about sorting the items and giving things up. Think of it as releasing them back into the world.

Once you're done sorting, it's time to think: Which of the clothes go to charity? Which ones get sold online? Which ones get given to friends and family? Which ones are you not sure about, and maybe you'd like to try them in front of a mirror one last time?

When you're finished, get back to your closet. Clean it. Make room for the returning tenants. Arrange it so that they're easy to see and reach.

It feels amazing, doesn't it? You're opening your own closet and it's like walking into a fancy shop where there's only pretty things that you, specifically you, really love, without any unwanted obstacles getting in the way.

Now, choose something to wear tonight, for fun, just to be happy and celebrate the new look of your wardrobe.

If you liked today's exercise, you might want to look up Marie Kondo, and her book, *The Life-Changing Magic of Tidying*. In the book, Kondo does a similar exercise, but includes all the clothes...and everything else in the house, up to the last scrap notebook. It's a great way to get a fresh start.

I hope you had fun today, and you feel you have the best wardrobe you've ever had, with only the things you really love, to wear every day.

Tomorrow, you are going to take the next step and decide what new clothes can come into your wardrobe.

DAY 19: CHOOSING NEW CLOTHES

Hello, beautiful!

First, let me congratulate you on completing the eighteenth day of the 30-day vegan beauty makeover and getting your wardrobe sorted. Elimination is always hard, but after you do it, it feels great, doesn't it?

This is the nineteenth day of the program and today, you're going shopping.

The aim is to bring home one and only one new item to your freshly sorted wardrobe. Why just one? When you buy something new, it's important to choose it just like you've chosen what to keep in your wardrobe. When only one item gets to win its ticket to go home with you, it will keep you focused. You will only choose what's best: it's a competition, and there's only one medal.

Dress to impress:
There are many, many ways to decide how to dress right. You will find plenty of advice on what to wear with what, what not to wear at all, and so on. So much, that it can really get confusing, because taste and fashion are different from place to place, and what works for others doesn't always work for you.

Question 1: What do you like?
This is the most important one: Only you know what really works for you, for your body shape and, even more importantly, for your personality. What clothes make you tick? Look at the things that you kept yesterday, and compare them with the things that you released. What's the difference? Maybe you find that you like strong colors. Maybe you like pastel. Maybe you like flowery clothes that make you feel like spring. Maybe you like contrasts, like wearing a bright scarf on top of a

dark sweater. What do you like?

Question 2: Whose style inspires you?
Think of someone whose style you like. Pick a celebrity who looks like you and also has an everyday style you would happily wear. This is a bit tricky. Most celebrities won't qualify - you want someone with similar hair, eyes, skin, and figure as you. They also have to be dressed in a style that you like, with clothes you can wear to work or for meeting friends (not their red-carpet items...). Look at different photos. Which items do you think would work well for you?

Also, think of people you know. Is there anyone whose style inspires you?

Question 3: What do you love about yourself?
Put on something very tight and look at yourself in the mirror. Pick three things that you really love about yourself. It could be your eyes, or your legs, or your curves. What are the most attractive parts of you that you want everyone to see? Which items in your wardrobe show them off? Maybe it's that scarf that brings out your eye color, or the tight-fitting jeans.

Question 4: What do you want people to see?

If you had to accentuate only one thing, what would it be?

Here's a winner's tip: The eye gets easily distracted. If you want something to really show, you don't want to shift the attention to other things. If you have a necklace you like, don't wear it with earrings (and vice versa) because the shine of the jewelry is too close and the eye would catch the whole instead of the item you want to show. The same is true for the body. If you're showing cleavage, or wearing a tight top, you want to combine that with a loose-fitting bottom, or a long skirt or pants. What do you want people to really see?

Question 5: What would you like to add?

This is the part where you're going to go shopping.

Go out there and get something really nice, something that makes you happy when you touch it, just like the clothes you decided to keep in your delightful new wardrobe yesterday.

When you are in the shop, ask for assistance. Find someone who is happy to give you tips about colors, or styles, or what would fit you best. Try their advice; see if you like it. Don't feel obligated to buy anything if you don't want to. Just have fun with it. See what you can learn.

I hope you have a great time today, getting connected to how you want to present yourself and your body, and find something new and beautiful to wear.

In the next two days, you are going to start getting ready for the most challenging week of the program, by learning about detox.

DAY 20: CLEANING THE BODY

Hello, beautiful!

First, let me congratulate you on completing the nineteenth day of the 30-day vegan beauty makeover and getting yourself something new and beautiful to wear. Have you worn it today already?

This is the twentieth day of the program and today and tomorrow, you're going to start preparing for the final and most challenging and rewarding week of the makeover, by learning about detox. You also have a new recipe, the Amazing Asian Radish Salad, which you will find at the end of the book, in the recipe section.

It's impossible to do a real natural makeover without learning how the body cleanses itself and rejuvenates. The more you know about your body, the more you'll be able to take good care of it, make healthy lifestyle choices, and protect it from any toxic environment.

The most basic part of understanding detox is knowing that there are four ways in and out of the body:

1. Skin
2. Breathing
3. Solids
4. Liquids

1) Skin:

Do you know how nicotine patches or birth control patches work? The skin absorbs the substances in the patch and these get into the bloodstream.

This process happens all the time. The skin absorbs what you put on it. Try mashing a banana or an avocado and creating a nice cream to put on. You'll see how, in a few minutes, the skin underneath will be soothed and refreshed.

The skin is also a way out of the body. When

you sweat, toxins come out of the body through the skin.

2) Breathing:

Here, we will include your ears, mouth, nose, throat, and lungs.

Breathing in nourishes you with vital oxygen, but chemicals in the air can also get in, and when you breathe out or cough, chemicals from the body come out. Do you remember walking by a place where the air was tight and polluted and then coughing heavily after that? That is how the breathing system cleans itself.

3) Solids:

The digestive system is the system we are the most used to thinking of, when considering the paths in and out of the body.

Every time you put something into your mouth, your body breaks it down and absorbs valuable nutrients. When it's done, it removes any remaining, unnecessary rubbish. This is also a way to remove toxins out of the body.

4) Liquids:

This one is a bit more complex to understand.

There are two fluids in the body: blood, which is pumped by the heart, and lymph, which flows using muscle movement.

Every cell in the body is like a little baby. It gets nutrients in through the blood, and toxins out through the lymph. The blood must always be kept clean and alkaline; the lymph is the acidic sewage. This is eventually filtered through the kidneys, and comes out of the body as liquid, when you go to the toilet.

The entire system that deals with this method of toxin removal is called the lymphatic system. It includes your lymph nodes, your kidneys, and your adrenal glands, which power the kidneys, and your bladder. It is a very complex sewage system, which keeps your body clean.

Since lymph in the body is moved by muscles, it's important to keep moving throughout the day.

I hope you feel you've learned something new and valuable, and gained a basic understanding of the four ways in and out of the body.

Okay, time for a treat! Head over to the recipe section and have a wonderful salad.

Tomorrow, you are going to go one step further and learn more about detox and cleansing.

DAY 21: DETOX

Hello, beautiful!

First, let me congratulate you on completing the twentieth day of the 30-day vegan beauty makeover and gaining valuable knowledge about your body! You are about to enter the final and most challenging week of the program.

This is the twenty-first day and today, you're going to learn what to expect when your body goes through a cleanse.

In the past twenty days, you've been eating healthy foods, reducing chemicals, building your self-love and happiness, relieving stress, and connecting to your natural, beautiful body. You've been learning how to be beautiful in so many ways. You are already feeling the powerful effects of the makeover, and you will at some point start experiencing detox symptoms.

1) What is detox?

Detox is the process in which the body rids itself of acids, toxins, and parasites.

Toxins and damaged cells can accumulate in the body. During detox, the body cleans them out and rebuilds internal tissue, cells, and organs. This is exactly the same as healing from an external or internal wound. As a result of detox, the body heals and symptoms are cured permanently. It's important to let the body clean itself, as far as it wants to.

2) What does detox feel like? What should you expect?

Remember the four ways in and out of the body? This is how the toxins are going to be cleaned from the system.

It can feel uncomfortable.

The body will use all four ways to clean itself. It will sneeze, sweat, and cough. It might raise a fever, go to the toilet very often, or have other flu-type symptoms, until it's clean, until what doesn't belong in the body gets out.

It's very important to rest and stay hydrated. Avoid heavy foods and chemicals. If you really feel that something is wrong, see a doctor. After all, not every discomfort is detox.

After the cleanse is complete, you will see a real change in the body. Wrinkles will disappear, nails and hair will be stronger, you'll have a lot more energy, physical activity will be easier, and you will be more focused. You will become more radiant, beautiful from the inside out.

3) How can you control detox?

You can bring up the pace or relax the detox by going up and down on the pyramid of foods:

At the top of the pyramid are the most nutrient-dense foods, which are herbs that grow in nature. You'll learn more about herbs on day 24.

Next, come the fruits, which as a frugivore species, are the most suitable for your metabolism. Bananas, apples, oranges, melons, cucumbers, tomatoes, etc. - anything that grows on plants, bears seeds, and has a high water content.

Below that are the vegetables. In colder countries where food has gone through refrigeration, and fruit has been depleted of nutrients, vegetables are important (but less detoxifying than fruits).

Below the vegetables are all other plants, including nuts and seeds, and foods that grow on or under the earth.

Then, come cooked foods. When a food is cooked above 42 degrees Centigrade or 108 Fahrenheit, enzymes and nutrients are destroyed, trans-fatty acids are created, and free radicals are formed. If you take an apple and you put it in the ground, you'll get an apple tree, but if you cook the apple, you'll destroy it. That is why fresh whole foods are higher on the pyramid than cooked foods.

Lowest on the food pyramid are processed foods and animal products, which are not detoxifying.

Going up on the detox pyramid creates stronger cleansing, with stronger symptoms.

Sometimes the symptoms are too hard, or you have another reason to stop the detox. If you want to reduce the detox, go downward in the pyramid. That's okay. Pick it back up tomorrow.

I hope you now feel more confident in your understanding of how the body cleanses itself and you are more ready for the final week of your beautiful makeover.

Tomorrow, you are going to have fun creating your own scent with essential oils.

DAY 22: SENSUAL SCENT

First, let me congratulate you on completing the twenty-first day of the 30-day vegan beauty makeover and learning all about detox.

This is the twenty-second day of the program and today, you're going to create your own fragrant stamp in the world, using essential oils. You also have a new recipe, the Magic Mediterranean Salad, which you will find at the end of the book, in the recipe section.

Creating your own blend of essential oils is very

easy. All you are going to need is 2–3 pure essential oils, a small empty bottle (about 50–100 ml) and a good carrier oil to blend them in. It's recommended that you use the grapeseed carrier oil from day 6.

The blend that you are going to make today can be used on your skin instead of perfume; on your hair, especially overnight - to give it both volume and moisture; and as a chemical-free deodorant.

Step 1) Shopping for Ingredients:
First, start by locating a good shop in your area that carries essential oils. It could be the pharmacy or the local health food store.

When you are there, ask to smell the pure (100%, non-diluted) essential oils. Treat this just like shopping for perfume. Make sure that you get something you really love. You can put a little bit on your finger, or bring some cotton pads with you to see what a few drops smell like.

There are plenty of essential oils to choose from, and a few carrier oils (my personal favorite is grapeseed oil, with its soft, sweet smell, which I also use as a makeup remover).

Some popular essential oils are: balsam fir, bergamot, cedarwood, chamomile, cinnamon, clove, frankincense, geranium, grapefruit, jasmine, lime, myrrh, neroli, patchouli, rose, sandalwood, tangerine, vanilla, vetiver, wild orange, and ylang ylang.

The oils will last for a long time. Some will last a few years at least. Some evaporate quickly, like jasmine, so make sure you get a good brand.

Step 2) Blending:

This is actually really easy. The aim here is to have about 2% of essential oils in the carrier oil.

1. First, write down the number of different essential oils you are going to use:

____________ scents

Example: ___4___ scents (lavender, patchouli, clove, vanilla)

2. Now, using a tablespoon, fill the empty bottle with your carrier oil, like grapeseed oil. Write down how many tablespoons you've used:

____________ tablespoons

Example: ___10__ tablespoons

3. Double the number of tablespoons and write it down – this will be the total number of essential oil

drops you will use:

___________ drops of essential oils.

Example: _______2x10__ = __20_ drops of essential oils.

4. Now, divide the last number by the number of different essential oil scents you bought. This will be the number of drops from each scent:

___________ drops each scent

Example: 20 drops of essential oils, divided by 4 scents = __5__ drops from each scent

After you've done it once, you won't need to calculate anymore. You'll get a feel for it.

Ok! Time to grab the dropper and make the mix.

I hope you have fun today, and you feel more connected to yourself and your beauty, with a nice new fragrant scent that's entirely your own.

Three days to a grape fast...

Okay, time for a treat! Head over to the recipe section and have a wonderful salad.

Tomorrow, you're having a makeup tutorial.

DAY 23: A DASH OF MAKEUP

Hello, beautiful!

First, let me congratulate you on completing the twenty-second day of the 30-day vegan beauty makeover and getting your very own beautiful scent.

This is the twenty-third day of the program and today you will have a makeup tutorial.

Makeup is one of the ways we express ourselves or augment our facial expressions and non-verbal messages. Of course, you always want to make sure that the ingredients you use are natural. This will also be an opportunity to use some of the new products you purchased on day 8.

Step 1) Facial Wash:
Start by washing your face with some nice warm water. Then, with cold water to close the pores. Dry with a fresh towel.

Step 2) Cream:
Once your face is dry, apply natural cream or a little bit of aloe vera, straight from a plant. Massage your skin while doing so, to increase circulation.

Step 3) Foundation:
The next step is putting on a base layer of foundation, to get an even skin color across the face. If you have very strong facial features, you might want to skip this step, or alternatively, do only this.

When applying foundation, make sure to use a shade that is similar to your natural tone, so that it isn't immediately noticeable. You want to give the impression of, "I am proud of how I look. I only use minimal makeup to accentuate what I already have." Spread the layer evenly.

You can do this step using your fingers, a large

brush, or a makeup sponge.

Step 4) Concealer:

When you are done with the foundation, carefully apply a thin layer of concealer in areas you want to cover (like that cute little mosquito bite behind the left cheek...). Then, use a bit under your eyes, on any area that is dark. Focus on the inner part of the eye, near the nose, and leave the outer part concealer-free. This will intensify the effect.

Also apply it on the top of the cheekbones, right below the eyes, to make your cheekbones look slightly higher.

You can do this step using your fingers, a small brush, or a makeup sponge. With some products, you can use the foundation itself, if it's light enough and has a strong texture, instead of purchasing a concealer.

Step 5) Blush:

The next step is to put some blush on. You don't actually have to use a special product for this. With most shades of lipstick, you can put a little bit of lipstick on your cheeks and spread it.

A small tip: the professional model-type look has

blush on the sides of the cheeks and up toward the cheekbones. You would get a much younger, rosy and energetic look if, instead, you don't apply blush on the sides at all, but put only a little bit on the front of the cheeks, under the eyes.

You can do this step using your fingers, a large brush, or a makeup sponge.

Step 6) Eye shadow (optional):
The next step is optional. For some people, a little bit of dark eye shadow accentuates the eyes without creating an unnatural dramatic look.

If you choose to do this, take a pencil and place it between the bottom of your nose and the outer end of your eyebrow. Apply the dark shadow only to the skin above the eye and below the pencil. Start by putting just a little bit, right on the crease. Gently blend it toward the eyebrow, keeping most of the color concentrated on the crease.

It's best to do this step using either your fingers, or a small brush with a sloped end.

Step 7) Either Lipstick or Eyeliner/Mascara:
Once you're done with the previous steps, you're going to make a choice between putting on lipstick or eyeliner. This is one of the best makeup

tips out there.

When you look at photos or videos of people, like on YouTube, in a magazine, in movies, or on television, you normally see a lot of makeup. Unfortunately, most people forget that these images are all flat - you cannot tell their depth. To get a good effect in an image, you have to use plenty of makeup, but this doesn't look good in real life.

In real life, people are three-dimensional. If you look at a magazine model, fresh from a photoshoot, she would look like she's wearing too much makeup, and you'd think she's overly done it.

For this reason, you want to accentuate only one part of your face, similarly to what you've done with clothing. Choose to put makeup on either the eyes or the lips.

If you've chosen the lips, apply a thin layer of lipstick or lip gloss and spread it evenly.

If you've chosen the eyes, apply a very thin layer of eyeliner, right on top of the eyelashes. This will be almost invisible and will create an illusion of thicker eyelashes. If you want the eyeliner to show, you can add a bit more to the outer half of the eye.

On the other hand, if you're going for a very natural look, you can choose to apply eyeliner only to the outer half.

Another natural-looking method for thicker eyelashes is wearing mascara without eyeliner. Mascaras are a little bit more concealed. Most men wouldn't notice a woman has mascara on, if she's not wearing eyeliner with it.

This is the end of the "natural look" makeup tutorial.

I hope you had a great time today, and have inspiration on how to bring out the best of you.

Two days to a grape fast...

Tomorrow, you are going to learn about the great benefits of herbs.

DAY 24: THE MAGIC OF HERBS

Hello, beautiful!

First, let me congratulate you on completing the twenty-third day of the 30-day vegan beauty makeover and getting creative with colors.

This is the twenty-fourth day of the program and today you have an extremely important lesson. So far, you've learned about the importance of your inner organs to your health and overall beauty. Today, you'll take it one step further and learn about herbs that can help you rebuild internal tissue.

This is also the day to start getting ready for the grape fast, which is on days 26 and 27, by purchasing 6 kilograms, or 13.2 pounds, of grapes.

Herbs are the strongest, most nutrient dense, of all foods. They are great for both strengthening the body, for building new cells and tissue, and for detoxification.

Let's have a look at some of the most common herbs, which you can find in the supermarket or at the corner Asian shop.

- Parsley: great for your kidneys. Has four times the iron per gram as red meat.
- Juniper berry: also good for the kidneys.
- Dandelion: great for your liver.
- Turmeric: also good for your liver, which creates, stores, and converts valuable chemicals for the whole body.
- Kelp and seaweed: great for your thyroid, which balances heat in the body.
- Fenugreek seeds: great for breaking mucus. When you get a cold, boil one teaspoon of fenugreek seeds in one cup of water for six minutes. Strain and drink; it's just like a warm cleansing tea and you'll immediately feel the difference.

- Aloe vera: great for putting on your skin, to nourish and alkalize it.
- Black Walnut hull and wormwood seed: great for killing parasites, including larger ones like worms and flukes. You can purchase a compound of them online in gelatin form (don't use during pregnancy or when breastfeeding).
- Pau D'Arco: also good for killing parasites.
- Cloves: great for destroying parasite eggs.
- Burdock root: helps remove acids from your body.
- Butcher's Broom: anti-inflammatory and good for your circulation.
- Chamomile: anti-inflammatory and good for your digestion.
- Comfrey Root: great for building strong connective tissue, which holds cells, organs, and glands together.
- Ginger: great for your digestion and for your circulation.
- Valerian: a natural calmer.
- He Shou Wu: an antioxidant, great for your hair.

Give yourself a treat today. Pick a few of these herbs and use them in a meal. Give your body these great nutrient foods, which you can easily get, and connect to the pharmacy of nature!

If you want to know more about herbs and how they connect to the functions of the body, a great book is *The Detox Miracle Sourcebook* by Robert Morse, whose interview you had on day 13.

I hope you enjoy a special nutrient-dense meal with lots of great herbs. It is a real treat.

One day to a grape fast...

Tomorrow, you are going to do a special exercise to connect to your dreams and inner desires.

DAY 25: KNOWING YOURSELF

Hello, beautiful!

First, let me congratulate you on completing the twenty-fourth day of the 30-day vegan beauty makeover and getting to know the beauty of herbs.

This is the twenty-fifth day of the program and today, you are going to do a special exercise to connect to your true self. You also have a new recipe, Cream of Celery Soup, which you will find at the end of the book, in the recipe section.

Tomorrow is going to be the first of the two-day grape fast, so now would be a good time to purchase 6 kilograms, or 13.2 pounds, of grapes, if you haven't had a chance to do so yet.

And now to self-discovery:

A lot of times, life brings us into a certain routine: a job, a career, a social circle, and a way of life. We get used to seeing things in a certain way. This is a good thing, as it gives us comfort. Unfortunately, it's possible to become too focused, and get lost in the routine. Certain wants, desires, and dreams might get moved aside and even forgotten.

It's very important to reconnect to your true self from time to time. Many times, when you rediscover what it is that you truly want, you will also discover that the changes you want to make are very minor.

I have coached people using the following exercise, called "Magic Wand." It works on releasing our limitations and exposing the true wishes that lie below.

Let's get started.

Question 2:

You are back to how you were before the previous question. Now, the magic wand is going to give you unlimited time. You will live forever. You have all the time in the world. What do you do?

____

____

____

____

____

____

____

____

Question 3:

You are back to how you were before the previous question. Now, the magic wand is going to give you a magical ticket. This magical ticket has two features.

1. Exactly one year from now, you will reappear here, just as you are at this moment. During that time, your life will go on, but right at the end of the year, you will be back here and now, and only you will remember what you'd done during this time. No one else will even know. There will be no traces or consequences of anything you do. You can go anywhere and do anything.

2. The ticket is also a card that can pay for anything, anywhere. You can see the world, live in a castle, start a business, or just lay on the beach. However, everything will be completely erased exactly one year from now, when you magically return to this moment.

What do you do?

Question 4:

You are back to how you were before the previous question. Now, the magic wand is going to give you a magical ring. When you wear this ring, no one will know what you're doing. It can happen right in front of them and they won't notice it. You can go anywhere in the world and come back and your friends will somehow not know about it at all. You can do whatever you want. No one will ever find out. What do you do?

____

____

____

____

____

____

____

____

____

____

____

So, what have you learned today? What are the things about yourself that surprised you? Did you discover anything you'd like to try? Maybe something you'd like to change?

From my experience, most people who have done this exercise got better connected to their inner desires, and they did change things afterward, but surprisingly not in the same way that they did in the exercise. This is more about possibilities, about releasing the boundaries and rules that you get used to. It's not about replacing the current way with the one discovered during the exercise, but rather about finding a good third way.

You can play this game with your friends and have fun. Only make sure to remind them that their answers are more about possibilities and they are not obligated to do anything that they say they want to do when they play the game.

In order for you to use this technique further to know yourself, and help those you play with, the following paragraphs will explain the inner workings of Magic Wand, so that you can use it to add new questions.

All the questions are really a variation of: "I have a limitation - what would I do if I didn't have this limitation?"

In the first question, the limitation was money. This is the easiest one to start with, since it's the subject that all of us are used to thinking of. When you first ask a person this question, they'd normally answer immediately that they'd like a vacation, or buy a large house, or do the kind of things you see on television. When you ask them what they'd do a year from now, that's when things get creative.

In the second question, the limitation was time. Again, one that many people think of on a regular basis, but here there is more space for creativity. This is important, as it frees the imagination for the next questions.

The third and fourth questions are more complex. Both of them target the limitation of pride. Pride comes from our sense of how people see us. "What will others think of what I do?" We have morals and rules based on this. But what if nobody knew what you were doing? What would you do then? What if the limitations of your current society, country, and friends were removed? What if your actions had no consequences?

Now that you understand how Magic Wand works, you can create your own questions. Think of something you want to do or have. Then find out what is stopping you by saying, "I wish I could do this, if only I had..." and complete the sentence with what's limiting you. Then create a Magic Wand question that removes the limitation.

For example: say that you currently have a lot of problems and you don't know where to start tackling them. Imagine the magic wand gives you a magical cube. Toss the cube, then look at the bottom. There you'll see the problem that must be solved first. Which one was it?

You will find that when you've done this exercise a few times, your answers won't look so different than the life you're already living. This is because with time, you will learn to make the changes you need to have and do the things that make you who you really are.

I hope you got a true connection to your inner wishes through this exercise, that you connected to your own flame, and your inner beauty.

Okay, time for a treat! Head over to the recipe section and have a wonderful soup.

Tomorrow, you are going to start the most challenging part of the makeover: the two-day grape fast. Good luck!

DAY 26: GRAPE FAST DAY 1

Hello, beautiful!

First, let me congratulate you on completing the twenty-fifth day of the 30-day vegan beauty makeover and getting in touch with your deepest desires.

This is the twenty-sixth day of the program and today you are about to enter the greatest challenge of all: the two-day grape fast.

I'll tell you a secret. Grape fasting is actually really easy. You won't feel tired or hungry. On the contrary, you'll have lots of energy and feel light and flowing. The only part that's hard is thinking about other foods. So, right now, decide that for two days, you don't have to think about foods. You are free of them. There are so many other interesting things in life. Think about those instead. Free space in your mind for other tasks. Watch a nice movie while nibbling grapes.

Before you begin this grape fast, there is one small preparation you should be aware of: on day 28 and 29, the two days right after the fast, you will time your food differently, to assist your body in filtering out toxins that were released through the grape fast. This is very important, to ensure these toxins move easily out of your body. On day 28, you will have a very early dinner, as early as 3 or 4 in the afternoon, and on day 29 you will have brunch instead of breakfast, at 9 or 10 in the morning. You'll read more about this on day 28.

Fasting is one of the most natural and easiest ways to clean the body of toxins. It's the shortest route in detox. There is a wide range of different types of fasting, each with different benefits. The grape fast is one of the most balanced of the mono-meal fasts, which are fasts where you only eat one food (mono means one). There are many cases of people who have done this for a few weeks to a few months (which requires supervision, and high quality organic grapes). My own personal experience was 13 days at most, under supervision.

The longest you can fast for a first time without supervision is 2–3 days. For that length of time, most people can successfully do almost any fast on their own.

During the fast, make sure to eat regularly. You will be eating 3 kilograms, or 6.5 pounds, of grapes per day, which would give you around 2,000 calories. You might want to make them into smoothies as you go along, which will make them easier to drink. If you feel that is too difficult, you can strain the smoothies and drink the grapes as a juice. It's only two days, and you don't need to worry about sugars when juicing for such a short period of time.

Eat as much and as often as you want. Don't think about what time of day you eat. Do what feels comfortable. You might be surprised to discover that you don't really feel much of a difference, despite eating in a different way.

At the end of the fast, you will notice changes. Your skin will be brighter and more shiny.

Wrinkles will soften and you will feel lighter and more vibrant. You might also find that cravings you previously found difficult to control are easier to handle or have disappeared entirely.

I wish you a happy and easy first day of fasting, with consistent energy and lightness.

Tomorrow, you are going to complete the fast and already experience some of its great benefits.

DAY 27: GRAPE FAST DAY 2

Hello, beautiful!

First, let me congratulate you on completing the first day of the two-day grape fast. Well done! One more day to go...

This is the second day of the fast.

You have probably already noticed the difference in the body, the lighter feeling. Perhaps you needed less sleep and experienced more energy in the morning.

Today, you're going to push it a little bit further

and end either late tonight, or tomorrow morning during breakfast.

There is a special task that you might want to do this evening. During fasting, many times you will experience clarity of thought and increased focus. This is because less of your energy is being used for digestion, so more was left for other uses. Unlike a normal meal, eating the same fruit over and over throughout the day is very easy on the stomach, since the speed and chemicals needed are consistent, and in addition, your mind is free from thoughts about food.

This evening, before going to sleep, write down your thoughts. Let them flow on the paper. See what lessons were awaiting you from this experience. You might find a deeper connection to things. You might also find that problems that previously burdened you now seem to be less important, and something far more valuable was awaiting your discovery underneath.

My inner thoughts and feelings - fasting journal:

____

Reut Barak

____

____

____

____

____

I hope you have a great experience with the fast.

If you are interested in fasting in general, or would like to attempt long-term fasting, I suggest you find a good professional, one who has supervised others during fasts, particularly if they come from a country or culture where fasting is prevalent (I once got help from a pharmacist from India).

Tomorrow, you are going to complete the cleanse by timing your food to get stronger kidney filtration.

DAY 28: DRY FASTING

Hello, beautiful!

First, let me congratulate you on completing the two-day grape fast. You are a star!

This is the twenty-eighth day of the program. Only two more days to go. Today, we are going to do something that's very important following a fast, which is to increase kidney filtration. This is done by timing your food slightly differently. You also have a new recipe for tomorrow morning, the Precious Peach Smoothie, which you will find at the end of the book, in the recipe section.

In the past two days, your body has worked

really hard, as thirty-seven trillion cells had a special opportunity to release toxins. This is a relief to the system as a whole, but just like every cleanup, somebody needs to take the rubbish out. In this case, the garbage masters are your kidney and adrenal glands, which make the kidneys work.

You might have noticed a little bit of darkness under your eyes this morning. This means that your kidneys and adrenals are working hard, as you may recall from the Chinese face maps. Today, you are going to ease their work, by changing the timing of your food.

Tonight, aim to have dinner very early, as early as 3 or 4 in the afternoon. Make sure you get enough liquids throughout the day. After you're done eating, do not consume any food or drink any liquids.

Then, tomorrow, have brunch instead of breakfast, at 9 or 10 in the morning. Don't eat or drink before that.

You must be wondering what is the benefit of this special timing. What you are about to experience is a very light "dry fast." It's called "dry," because no liquids go through the system. This is the highest form of fasting, and the one that gives your entire system the most rest. It's practiced in different religions, as a form of both physical and spiritual cleanse.

You might know people who don't like to eat or drink during most hours of the day, and their bodies naturally get dry fasts without them even noticing this.

Your aim is to get around 18 hours of dry fasting. During these hours, try to also get rest. The purpose of what you are doing is to give more power to the kidneys and adrenals, so that the toxins come out of your body more easily.

Make sure to get lots of sleep tonight.

Tomorrow morning, you might notice a change when you go to the toilet, as acids get released out of your system. You will probably feel very light and energized after that.

During the 18 hours, only drink if you feel extreme thirst, or if you're under the weather and you happen to get a fever.

And most importantly, plan a wonderful fruit brunch for tomorrow. Fruit is the way to break a fast, plus you deserve a treat! There's a fresh new smoothie recipe for you here, which comes tomorrow. Why not check the ingredients now so that you are prepared?

I hope you have a restful evening and a wonderful brunch tomorrow.

Tomorrow, you are going to take a step back and have a night out.

DAY 29: A NIGHT OUT

Hello, beautiful!

First, let me congratulate you on completing the twenty-eighth day of the 30-day vegan beauty makeover and getting through all the fasting! You are amazing. You have done something for yourself that so few people would do.

This is the second-to-last day of the program and today, you're going out!

Today, you also have the new recipe, the Precious Peach Smoothie, which you will find at the end of the book, in the recipe section.

It's time to put everything you've learned

together, but first, have yourself an amazing tasty smoothie for brunch, to break your dry fast; hydrate your body and fill it with loving nutrients. You deserve it.

Once you're done, start getting ready, because tonight you are going out. You're going to pick a nice restaurant where you can eat or do a takeaway of healthy, vegan, gluten – free foods, preferably from the raw menu. Give yourself a treat. Better yet, share it with friends.

When you are preparing, take your time. Pick something from your newly organized wardrobe, maybe that new item that you bought. Do your hair, your nails, and your eyebrows. Brush your skin. Before the shower, do a bit of a wild dance and then shower with natural soap and shampoo and put on natural makeup. Do an oil pull.

Then, when you go out, tell your friends about the great journey you've made, especially the last two days of fasting. Share it proudly. Socially sharing the journey is the best way to get the support that you need around you to ensure the new ways you've learned this last month stay with you. Be ready - they will probably ask a lot of questions, considering how much you glow!

Okay, time for a treat! Head over to the recipe section and have a wonderful smoothie.

I wish you a wonderful night out. You've made a long journey and you deserve your party.
Tomorrow is the last day, and it's going to be your vegan beauty celebration.

DAY 30: A VEGAN CELEBRATION

Hello, beautiful!

First, let me congratulate you on completing the journey. It's been a great month and you have made such a huge difference in such a short time.

You are a brave and beautiful woman, with a magnificent, dazzling soul. Few would have done all that you have!

Today's recipe will be a celebration of raw vegan sushi, which you will find at the end of the book, in the recipe section.

But before we get to it, let's do two things. First,

you're going to look at the amazing journey you have made, and second, you're going to find one thing from a previous day that you would like to repeat, or something you might have missed, and do that today. Today is all about getting a feeling of completion.

In the past thirty days, you have changed your lifestyle, gained knowledge, and gotten to know yourself as you never did before.

You learned how to take great care of yourself and your body. You've made your skin, hair, nails, eyebrows, and teeth look amazing. You've given your wardrobe a makeover. You've cleaned up your cosmetics and learned how to wear your makeup to look naturally glamorous. You've made your own blend of essential oils.

You've learned to relax, rest, and replenish your energy, sleep well, and release stress. You've gotten to know your body, how to take care of it and protect it, how to make it shine from the inside out and reverse the effects of time and the environment. You've learned about detox, how the body works and how to cleanse it. You've mastered kitchen herbs and learned how to combine your foods. You've done two days of fasting!!!

You got to connect to nature, and to your own

body through movement and through dancing.

You've gotten to know yourself, and worked on your self-esteem. You connected to your dreams and inner desires.

You've learned thirteen new smoothie, salad, noodles, wraps, soup, and sushi recipes.

And you've shared your experience with others.

You've done a huge transformation, and it is going to remain with you for the rest of your life.

Keep learning. Keep getting to know your beautiful self and your amazing body. It's a precious gift.

Look back at the things that you have written during the exercises you've done on days 7, 11, 25, and 27. See what a great journey you've made. Keep them. A year from now, look at them again. See how this experience has shaped you.

The secret to vitality, youthfulness, and health is in you. Only you know and feel your body from the inside. Keep searching for ways to connect to it. It's the most important thing you have in life. Share what you learn. Help others.

Before we part to make the sushi, I'd like to remind you of a quote you've learned on day 7:

"Be the flame, not the moth!"

By now, surely, you have found the things that make you who you are. You have found your inner and outer beauty and your confidence. Treasure those. Be a light to others. We'll all be watching you with pride.

RECIPES

RECIPE INDEX

DARING DILL SMOOTHIE

Preparation time: 5 minutes
Serves Two

Ingredients:

1 cup dill

2 cucumbers

the juice of 3 lemons

¼ cup mint

1 tablespoon rosemary

1 teaspoon tarragon

1 teaspoon oregano

½ teaspoon nutmeg powder

½ teaspoon paprika

Instructions:

In a food processor or high-speed blender, blend all ingredients until very smooth (you can leave out a few chopped vegetables for decoration).

Pour into glasses and serve.

YouTube Video for this recipe:
https://youtu.be/Q35Vw6l7BNM

Recipe source: The book, *100 Smoothies* (Raw Munchies Cookbooks Book 2): 100 raw vegan exotic smoothies, great for detox, and ready in 5 minutes.

TRADITIONAL PESTO NOODLES

Preparation time: 30 minutes
Waiting time: 20–40 minutes
Serves Two

Noodles:

6 zucchini
3 tablespoons cold-pressed olive oil
3 tablespoons coconut aminos
pinch salt

Pesto:

6 cups fresh basil leaves
3 teaspoons cold-pressed olive oil
1 ½ cups pine nuts
¾ cup walnuts
2 teaspoons garlic powder
pinch salt

Instructions:

Noodles:

Using a spiralizer julienne blade or a julienne
peeler, spiralize zucchini into noodles.

Mix well with olive oil, coconut aminos, and salt, and let the mixture stand for 20–40 minutes, to soften the noodles into a supple pasta-like texture. Once the Noodles are softened, remove the liquids.

Pesto:
In a food processor or high-speed blender, blend the Pesto ingredients until smooth.
Mix with the Noodles and serve.

Recipe source: The book, *30 Noodles* (Raw Munchies Cookbooks Book 3): 30 easy raw vegan noodle recipes with delicious popular spaghetti and pasta dishes.

CREATIVE COLORS OF THE RAINBOW SALAD

Preparation time: 30 minutes
Serves Two

Ingredients:

1 avocado

1 tomato

½ yellow bell pepper

½ cauliflower

½ red cabbage

the juice of 2 lemons

1 handful sunflower seeds

Instructions:

Chop avocado, tomato, pepper, and cauliflower into large pieces and slice the cabbage thin, to create a variety of textures.

Mix with the lemon juice and sunflower seeds and serve fresh.

Recipe source: The book, *50 Salads* (Raw

Munchies Cookbooks Book 4): 50 famous raw vegan salads from world cuisine, for quick, easy, and healthy meals.

MEGA MORNING GLORY SMOOTHIE

Preparation time: 5 minutes
Serves Two

Ingredients:

3 cups strawberries

3 cups grapes

1 mango

1 apple

1 banana

Instructions:

In a food processor or high-speed blender, blend all ingredients until very smooth (you can leave out a few chopped fruit for decoration).

Pour into glasses and serve.

Recipe source: The book, *100 Smoothies* (Raw Munchies Cookbooks Book 2): 100 raw vegan exotic smoothies, great for detox, and ready in 5 minutes.

MAGICAL MANGO BERRY SALAD

Preparation time: 30 minutes
Serves Two

Ingredients:

1 mango
1 cup blueberries
2 cups strawberries
6 bananas

Instructions:

Chop the fruit rough, to create a variety of textures. Mix and serve fresh.

Recipe source: The book, *50 Salads* (Raw Munchies Cookbooks Book 4): 50 famous raw vegan salads from world cuisine, for quick, easy, and healthy meals.

DARK DREAM SMOOTHIE

Preparation time: 5 minutes
Serves Two

Ingredients:

1 cup blackberries
2 cups strawberries
6 bananas
1 teaspoon alcohol-free vanilla extract

Instructions:

In a food processor or high-speed blender, blend all ingredients until very smooth (you can leave out a few chopped fruit for decoration).

Pour into glasses and serve.

Recipe source: The book, *100 Smoothies* (Raw Munchies Cookbooks Book 2): 100 raw vegan exotic smoothies, great for detox, and ready in 5 minutes.

LETTUCE WRAPS

Preparation time: 15 minutes
Serves Two

Leaves:

10–12 large lettuce leaves

Vegetables:

½ red pepper

½ cup chives

2 cups bean sprouts

1 tablespoon sesame oil

1 tablespoon coconut aminos

1 teaspoon maple syrup

½ teaspoon apple cider vinegar

½ teaspoon ginger

½ teaspoon nutmeg

½ teaspoon paprika

½ teaspoon 5 spice

Instructions:

Chop pepper and chives and mix with the rest of the Vegetables ingredients.

Carefully place in lettuce and roll, closing with a toothpick

YouTube Video for this recipe:
https://youtu.be/J_BsDhYxmEw

Recipe source: Raw Munchies introductory recipes on www.rawmunchies.org/recipes

FRESH STYLE PAD THAI NOODLES

Preparation time: 30 minutes
Waiting time: 20–40 minutes
Serves Two

Noodles:

2 zucchini
1 tablespoon cold-pressed olive oil
1 tablespoon coconut aminos
pinch salt

Dressing:

½ cup chives
½ red bell pepper
the juice of 1 lemon
½ tablespoon freshly grated ginger root
1 tablespoon coconut aminos
1 tablespoon cold-pressed sesame oil
½ tablespoon maple syrup

Vegetables:

1 carrot

4 radishes

1 cup bean sprouts

Garnish:

fresh coriander

Instructions:

Noodles

Using a spiralizer julienne blade or a julienne peeler, spiralize zucchini into noodles.

Mix well with olive oil, coconut aminos, and salt and let the mixture stand for 20–40 minutes, to soften the noodles into a supple pasta-like texture. Once the Noodles are softened, remove the liquids.

Dressing

In a food processor or high-speed blender, blend the Dressing ingredients until smooth.

Vegetables

Using a spiralizer julienne blade or a julienne peeler, spiralize carrot into noodles, and slice the radishes thinly. Mix with bean sprouts.

Mix Vegetables and Dressing. Pour over Noodles.

Garnish
Garnish with freshly chopped coriander.

Recipe source: The book, *30 Noodles* (Raw
Munchies Cookbooks Book 3): 30 easy raw vegan
noodle recipes with delicious popular spaghetti
and pasta dishes.

AMAZING ASIAN RADISH SALAD

Preparation time: 30 minutes
Serves Two

Ingredients:

2 cups radish
1 cucumber
1 avocado
¼ cup scallions
the juice of 2 lemons
½ teaspoon freshly grated ginger root
½ teaspoon cold-pressed sesame oil
½ teaspoon maple syrup

Instructions:

Using a spiralizer julienne blade or a julienne peeler, cut radish and cucumber into long, thin slices. Chop avocado and scallions.

Mix with the rest of the ingredients and serve fresh.

YouTube Video for this recipe:
https://youtu.be/ZxRWrCMifNY

Recipe source: The book, *50 Salads* (Raw Munchies Cookbooks Book 4): 50 famous raw vegan salads from world cuisine, for quick, easy, and healthy meals.

MAGIC MEDITERRANEAN SALAD

Preparation time: 30 minutes
Serves Two

Ingredients:

2 bell peppers in different colors

2 small cucumbers

2 tomatoes

½ onion

the juice of 1 lemon

1–2 tablespoons cold-pressed olive oil

pinch salt

Instructions:

Chop peppers, cucumbers, tomatoes, and onion into thin slices, to create an even texture.

Mix with the rest of the ingredients and serve fresh.

Recipe source: The book, *50 Salads* (Raw Munchies Cookbooks Book 4): 50 famous raw vegan salads from world cuisine, for quick, easy, and healthy meals.

CREAM OF CELERY SOUP

Preparation time: 15 minutes
Serves Two

Soup:

6 long celery ribs
½ cup chopped dill
the juice of 1 lemon
2 tablespoons cold-pressed olive oil
2 tablespoons rosemary
1 teaspoon nutmeg
1 teaspoon paprika
1 cup water
pinch garlic powder
pinch salt

Garnish:

chili flakes
chopped chives

Instructions:

Soup
In a food processor or high-speed blender, blend

all Soup ingredients until smooth.

Carefully heat to 108 degrees Fahrenheit (42 degrees Celsius), using a thermometer to check and ensure the temperature doesn't go higher.

Garnish

Garnish the soup with chili flakes and chopped chives, and serve warm.

Recipe source: The book, *Mission Raw* (Raw Munchies Cookbooks Book 1): 30 raw vegan recipes in 30 days.

PRECIOUS PEACH SMOOTHIE

Preparation time: 5 minutes
Serves Two

Smoothie:

5–6 peaches

1–2 cups strawberries

the juice of 7 oranges

1 teaspoon alcohol-free vanilla extract

½ teaspoon almond extract

Garnish:

sprinkle coconut flakes

Instructions:

In a food processor or high-speed blender, blend all ingredients until very smooth (you can leave out a few chopped fruit for decoration).

Pour into glasses, garnish with coconut flakes, and serve.

Recipe source: The book, *100 Smoothies* (Raw Munchies Cookbooks Book 2): 100 raw vegan exotic smoothies, great for detox, and ready in 5 minutes.

MEGA SUSHI

Preparation time: 20 minutes
Serves Two

Rice:

1 parsnip

the juice of ½ lemon

1 teaspoon freshly grated ginger root

1 teaspoon cold-pressed sesame oil

½ teaspoon maple syrup

½ teaspoon apple cider vinegar

½ teaspoon nutmeg

½ teaspoon ginger powder

Vegetables:

1 avocado

½ bell pepper

½ small cucumber

2–3 radishes

Sushi Sheets

3–4 untoasted nori sheets

Coating:

1 avocado

Sauce:

2 tablespoons coconut aminos

1 teaspoon maple syrup

½ teaspoon cold-pressed sesame oil

Decoration:

sesame seeds

Instructions:

Rice

Chop the parsnip. In a food processor, pulse until you reach rice consistency. Mix with the rest of the Rice ingredients.

Vegetables

Chop vegetables into thin, long slices.

Sushi Sheet

Wet a 3-inch (7 ½-centimeter) rectangle section across the nori sheet and place a Rice portion on it. Place Vegetables on top of the Rice and roll slowly, closing the sheet. Before reaching the end of the sheet, wet the top inch (2 ½ centimeter) of the sheet, to ensure the sushi remains closed.

Coating

Slice the avocado into halves, and remove the kernel. Using a large spoon, remove the inner section from the peel.

Turn the avocado over, and using a vegetable peeler, create thin slices. Wrap the sushi with the avocado slices.

Cut the sushi into bite-size pieces.

Sauce and Decoration

Mix Sauce ingredients and spread over the sushi, decorating with sesame seeds.

Recipe source: The book, *Mission Raw* (Raw Munchies Cookbooks Book 1): 30 raw vegan recipes in 30 days.

MORE RECIPES

The recipes in this book were provided courtesy of the RawMunchies© Cookbook Series.

You can find more free recipes here:
www.rawmunchies.org

RawMunchies.org
...it's a whole new way of cooking!

A quick guide to the books in the series is found on the next pages:

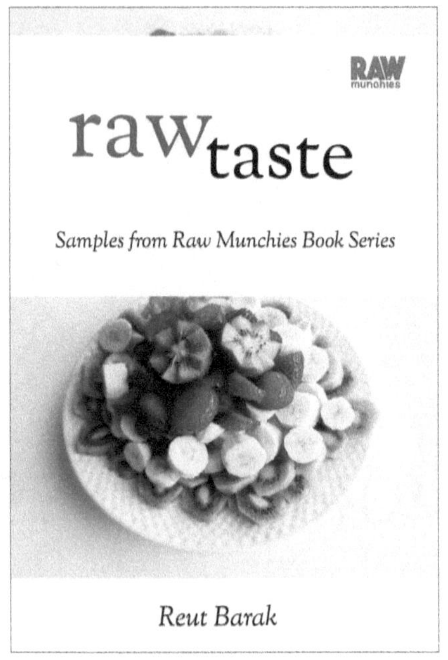

Free. All recipes have videos!

Downloadable on RawMunchies.org when joining the mailing list.

15 recipes from the books in the Raw Munchies series:

Precious Princess Smoothie
Playful Persimmon Smoothie
Orbit Orange Smoothie

Wicked Witches Brew
Pink Panda Smoothie
Daring Dill Smoothie
Overjoyed Olives and Corn Salad
Loving Lettuce with Guacamole Dressing
Amazing Asian Radish Salad
Bring-it-on Banana Kiwi Salad
Kelp Noodles, Farfalle
Meat Balls
Spicy Chicken Curry
Zucchini Crust Pizza

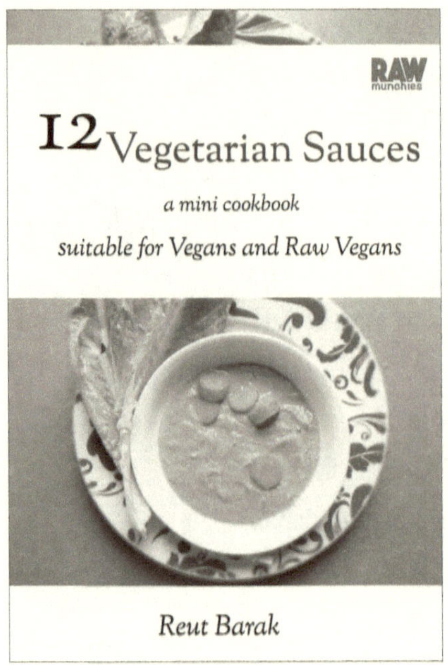

£0.99 or $1.50 on Amazon and online sellers.

A mini-cookbook - Suitable for Vegans and Raw Vegans (Raw Munchies Cookbooks) – available in E-book format:

A great companion to salads, noodles, desserts and party dips, this book is a perfect mini-cookbook for healthy foodies. All recipes are suitable for vegetarians, vegans, and raw vegans. There are also links to more free recipes, recipe ideas, and videos.

Book page and purchase links:
http://rawmunchies.org/12-sauces/

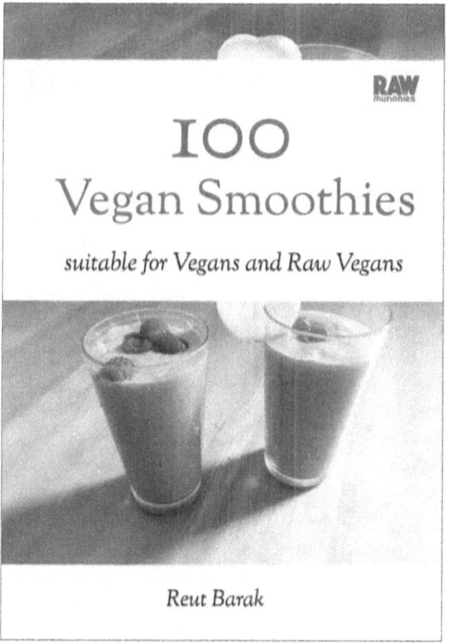

Quick and easy, energetic and mouth-watering smoothies. This book is all about health and ultra-detox. Simple food combining, and few

ingredients - a great way to have a quick, delicious meal, full of energy and ready in seconds.

100 recipes for a colorful adventure.

It's a whole new way of cooking!

Book page and purchase links:
http://rawmunchies.org/100-smoothies/

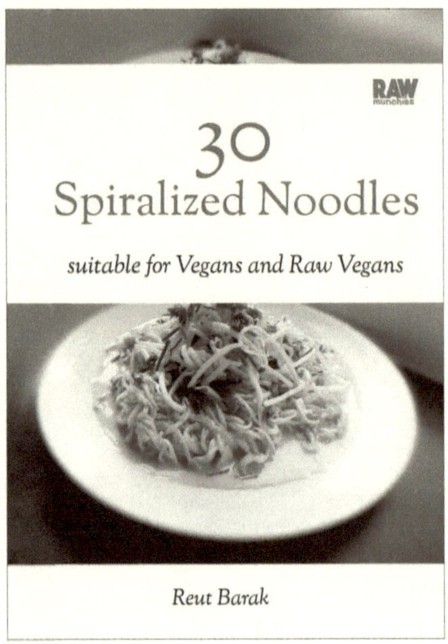

Easy pasta and noodles, featuring some of the most popular pasta and spaghetti recipes. This book has both regular and ultra-detox recipes - a great way to have a quick, impressive healthy meal.

30 recipes for 30 days of a spiralizing adventure. It's a whole new way of cooking!

Book page and purchase links:
http://rawmunchies.org/30-noodles/

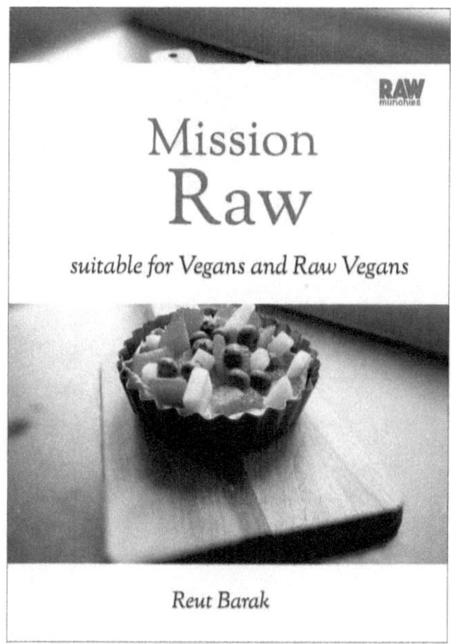

Delicious raw vegan versions of popular recipes. For everyone who wants a healthier pizza, burgers, sushi, and gourmet recipes - a great way to have a guilt-free, gluten-free, healthy meal.

30 recipes for 30 days of raw adventure.

It's a whole new way of cooking!

Book page and purchase links:
http://rawmunchies.org/mission-raw/

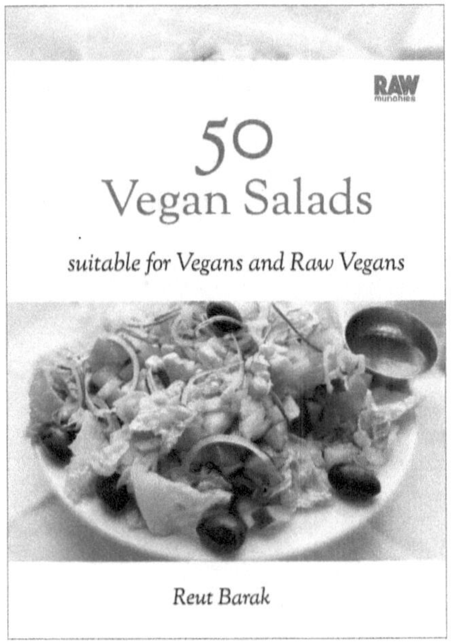

Quick, easy, and healthy recipes, with famous salads from world cuisine. This book has both regular and ultra-detox recipes - a great way to have a large, delicious meal or side dish, full of healthy nutrients and ready in minutes.

50 recipes for a crunchy adventure.

It's a whole new way of cooking!

Book page and purchase links:
http://rawmunchies.org/50-salads/

APPENDIX - MAKEUP TOXINS TO AVOID

Below is an alphabetical list of toxins found in makeup, compiled from different websites that specialize in tracking chemicals in cosmetics.

It's always best to keep looking up toxins online on a regular basis, because new chemicals are introduced every day.

1,4-dioxane
Acrylates
Benzophenone & Related Compounds (BHA)
BHA And BHT

Butylated Compounds

Carbon Black

DEA-related Ingredients

Diazolidinyl Urea

Dibutyl Phthalate

Ethanolamine Compounds (MEA, DEA, TEA)

Ethoxylated Ingredients

Ethyl

Formaldehyde

Formaldehyde-releasing Preservatives

Fragrance

Glycerin

Homosalate

Hydroquinone

Imidazolidinyl Urea

Lauramide DEA

Lead And Other Heavy Metals

Mercury

Methyl

Methylisothiazolinone

Methylchloroisothiazolinone

Mica

Nail Polish Removers

Nanomaterials

Nitrosamines

Octinoxate

P-phenylenediamine

PABA

Parabens Butyl

Parfum (aka Fragrance)

Peg Compounds

Petrolatum

Petroleum Jelly

Phenoxyethanol

Phthalates

Polyacrylamide

Polytetrafluoroethylene (PTFE, aka Teflon)

Preservatives

Propyl

Propylene Glycol

PVP/VA Copolymer

Quaternium-15

Red List

Resorcinol

Retinol And Retinol Compounds

Siloxanes

Sodium Laureth

Lauryl Sulfate (SLES/SLS)

Stearalkonium Chloride

Styrene Acrylates Copolymer

Synthetic Musks

Talc

Titanium Dioxide

Toluene

Triclosan

Triethylolamine

Coal Tar Dyes: P-phenylenediamine and colors

Listed as "ci" followed by a five digit number